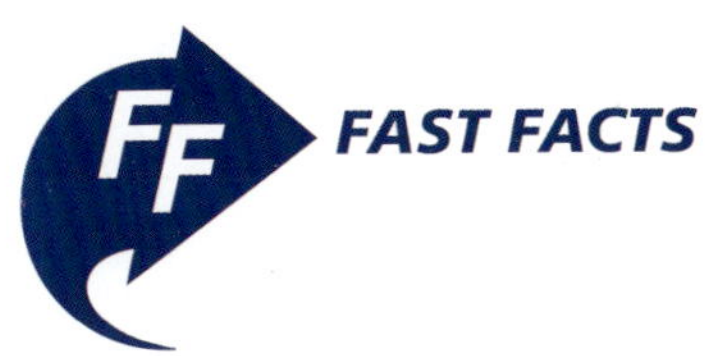

Perioperative Pain

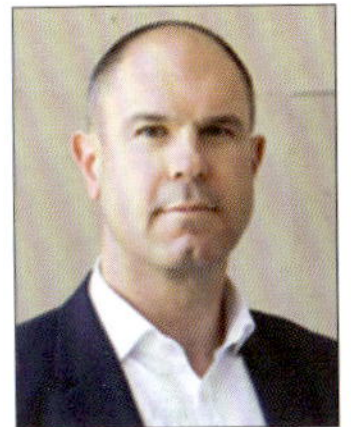

Matthew Brown MD (Res) MRCS FRCA FFPMRCA
Consultant in Pain Medicine and Anaesthetics
The Royal Marsden Hospital, and Honorary
Associate Faculty, The Institute of Cancer
Research, London, UK

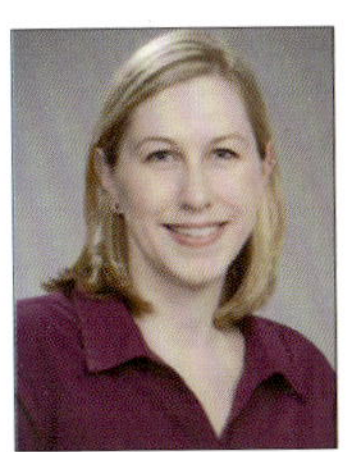

Katherin Peperzak MD
Assistant Professor
Department of Anesthesiology and Pain Medicine
University of Washington
Seattle, USA

Declaration of Independence

This book is as balanced and as practical as we can make it.

Ideas for improvement are always welcome: feedback@fastfacts.com

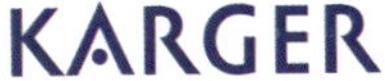

Fast Facts: Perioperative Pain
First published 2021

S. Karger Publishers Ltd, Elizabeth House, Queen Street,
Abingdon, Oxford OX14 3LN, UK
Tel: +44 (0)1235 523233

Book orders can be placed by telephone or email, or via the website.
Please telephone +41 61 306 1440 or email orders@karger.com
To order via the website, please go to karger.com

A CIP record for this title is available from the British Library.

ISBN: 978-3-318-06877-1

Brown M (Matthew)
Fast Facts: Perioperative Pain/
Matthew Brown, Katherin Peperzak

Medical illustrations by Graeme Chambers, Belfast, UK.
Typesetting by Amnet, Chennai, India.
Printed in the UK with Xpedient Print.

This edition has been supported by an independent educational grant from Heron Therapeutics.

For Henry, Amelie and Katharine (MB)

Thank you Chet, Paxton and Parker (KP)

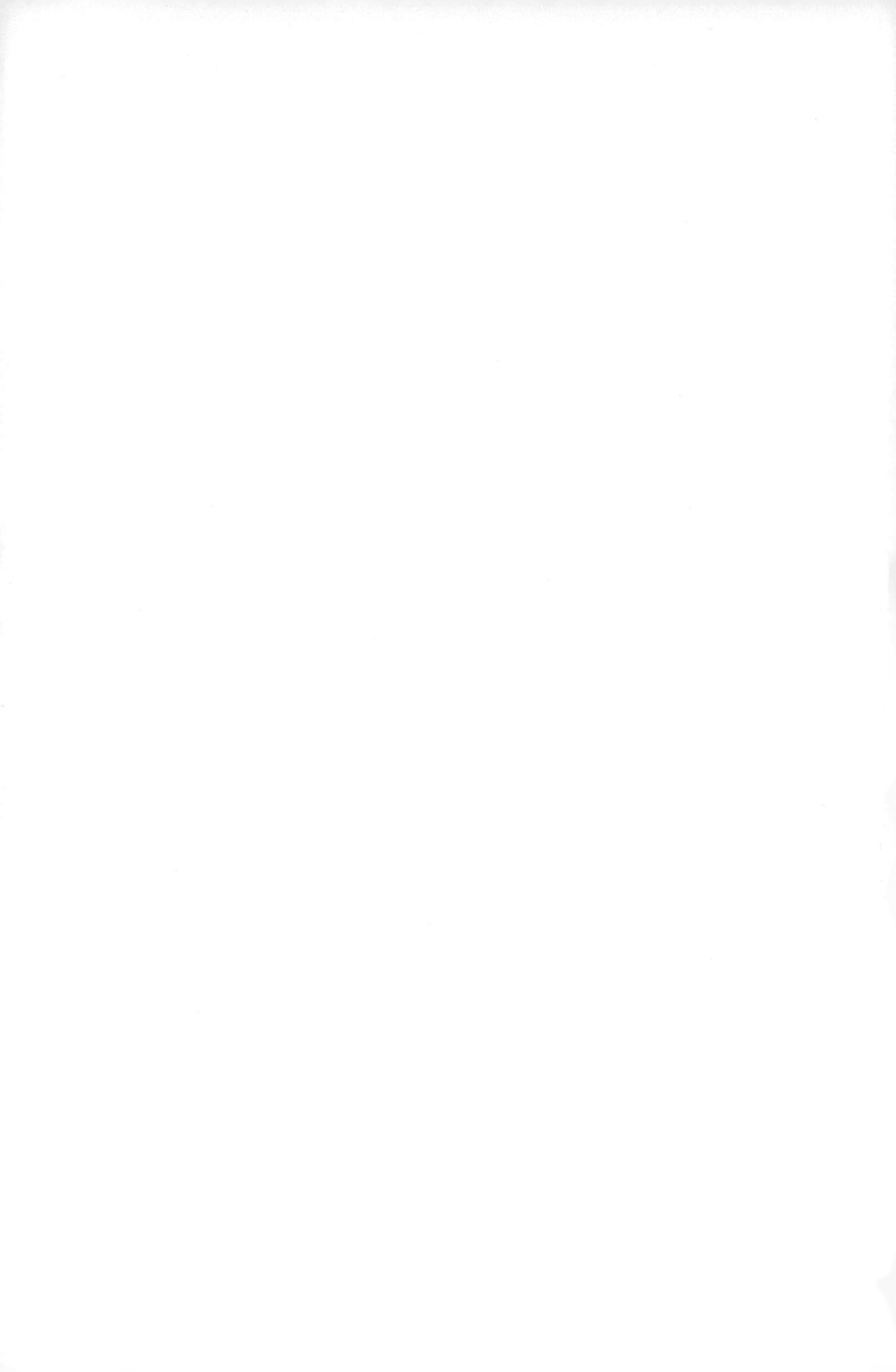

List of abbreviations

ACT: acceptance commitment therapy

ADD: assessment of discomfort in dementia

AMPA: α-amino-3-hydroxy-5-methyl-4-isoxazolepropionic acid

ANI: analgesia nociception index

CABG: coronary artery bypass grafting

CIWA: Clinical Institute Withdrawal Assessment for Alcohol

CNPI: checklist of nonverbal pain indicator

COPD: chronic obstructive pulmonary disease

COX: cyclo-oxygenase

CPOT: critical-care pain observation tool

CSE: combined spinal epidural

DSM: *Diagnostic and Statistical Manual of Mental Disorders*

ECG: electrocardiogram

ERAS: enhanced recovery after surgery

FLACC: face, legs, activity, cry, consolability

GABA: γ-aminobutyric acid

GFR: glomerular filtration rate

HIV: human immunodeficiency virus

HRV: heart rate variability

IASP: International Association for the Study of Pain

IV: intravenous

MAT: medication-assisted therapy

NAN: nociception–antinociception

NMDA: *N*-methyl-D-aspartate

NO: nitric oxide

NoL: nociception level (index)

NRS: numerical rating scale

NSAID: non-steroidal anti-inflammatory drug

OBAT: office-based addiction treatment (program)

OUD: opioid use disorder

PCA: patient-controlled analgesia

PCEA: patient-controlled epidural anesthesia

PKC: protein kinase C

PPSP: persistent postsurgical pain

PRD: pupil reflex dilation

PTSD: post-traumatic stress disorder

SAMHSA: Substance Abuse and Mental Health Services Administration

SBIRT: screening, brief intervention and referral to treatment (program)

SUD: substance use disorder

TENS: transcutaneous electrical nerve stimulation

TRPV1: transient receptor potential cation channel subfamily V member 1

VAS: visual analog scale

WMA: western medical acupuncture

Introduction

The importance of effective and safe pain management in the perioperative period has never been greater. The populations we serve as clinicians are rapidly changing, with increases in age, frailty and complexity of comorbidities. When these factors are considered in combination with socioeconomic issues, such as the 'opioid crisis' and budgetary constraint, it is clear that the challenges of providing a high-quality perioperative experience are extensive.

Attention has recently focused on the benefits of ensuring that pain in surgical patients is managed in an effective and compassionate fashion. From reduced postsurgical complications and minimization of hospital length of stay to improved patient satisfaction, these benefits are numerous and multidimensional. There have also been huge advances in the way in which we manage the perioperative pathway, both technical and organizational, as well as greater understanding of the underlying pathophysiology of pain states. Innovation in point-of-care imaging techniques, drug delivery, data science and patient engagement have all incrementally expanded the repertoire of the pain specialist.

Fast Facts: Perioperative Pain provides a succinct and accessible guide to the practice of perioperative pain management, covering the complete surgical journey from the preoperative assessment phase through to postoperative management. Consideration is given to our underlying understanding of the science of acute pain and how to assess it, as well as detailing the approaches – medical and non-medical – to managing acute pain and the evidence available to support these interventions. In addition, the phenomenon of persistent postsurgical pain is addressed, with an outline of its features, risk factors and potential preventive measures.

We trust that our book will prove a valuable resource for all multidisciplinary team members who encounter surgical patients in pain during the course of their work.

1 Pain mechanisms

The International Association for the Study of Pain (IASP) defines pain as 'An unpleasant sensory and emotional experience associated with, or resembling that associated with, actual or potential tissue damage.'[1] Acute pain as it relates to postoperative care is pain that is temporally related to a specific procedure and expected to reduce during an appropriate period of healing.[2,3] Social, cultural and personality factors may affect a patient's perception and response to pain, but generally acute pain responds well to treatment with analgesics and treatments targeted to the precipitating cause.

Pain can be classified in many different ways based on time course, mechanism or etiology (Table 1.1). One common categorization is to differentiate between nociceptive and non-nociceptive pain.[4]

Nociceptive pain

Somatic nociceptive pain is typically described as sharp, dull or aching. It is often worsened with movement and improved with rest. It tends to be localized and associated with an underlying lesion.

Specific examples of nociceptive pain include postsurgical pain, musculoskeletal pain and arthritic pain. Visceral nociceptive pain is less well localized and may be described as deep cramping or squeezing pain. It may be associated with autonomic sensations such as nausea, vomiting and diaphoresis. Patterns of pain referral exist, such as shoulder pain produced by diaphragmatic irritation following laparoscopic surgery.[5]

Mechanistically, nociceptive pain begins with a noxious stimulus (mechanical, thermal or chemical) that activates peripheral nociceptors and sends impulses along myelinated Aδ and unmyelinated C fibers to the spinal cord. These fibers synapse in the dorsal horn of the spinal cord before ascending to the thalamus, hypothalamus, reticular system and cortex of the brain, where the emotional and stress responses to pain are regulated (Figure 1.1).

TABLE 1.1

Potential ways of classifying pain

Time course

- Acute (<3 months)
- Subacute (≥6 weeks, <3 months)
- Chronic (≥3 months)
- Episodic

Etiology

- Cancerous
- Ischemic
- Postoperative
- Injury
- 'Cross-talk' between sympathetic and sensory neurons

Type of injured tissue

- Nociceptive
- Neuropathic
- Visceral
- Somatic

Intensity

- Mild
- Moderate
- Severe

Inferred mechanism

- Tissue damage
- Inflammation
- Central sensitization of nociceptors
- Nerve-damage-triggered neuroplasticity changes
- Brain neuroplasticity changes
- Loss of inhibition
- Glia-derived neural sensitization

In general, postoperative pain includes at least some component of nociceptive pain, as the nervous system is perceiving tissue damage from the procedure itself or an injury prompting a procedure to be performed.[6,7]

Potentiation. Following tissue or nerve damage, central potentiation occurs when peripheral nociceptors become sensitized in response to the accumulation of various endogenous chemicals and inflammatory mediators, such as bradykinin, prostaglandins,

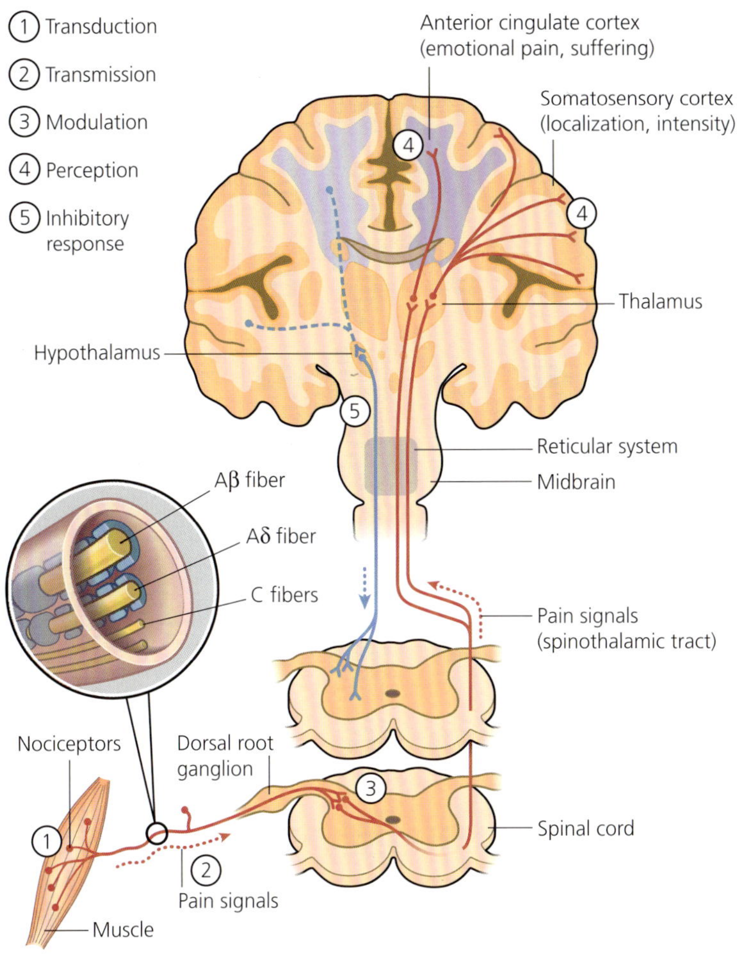

Figure 1.1 Nociceptive pathways. Nociceptive pain does not rely solely on passive transduction of pain signals; it also involves complex processing resulting in amplification and inhibition of noxious input.

histamine and interleukins (Figure 1.2). As pain persists, this sensitization and heightened afferent activity leads to chemical and anatomic reorganization in the spinal cord itself. In turn, this may lead to long-term central potentiation characterized by

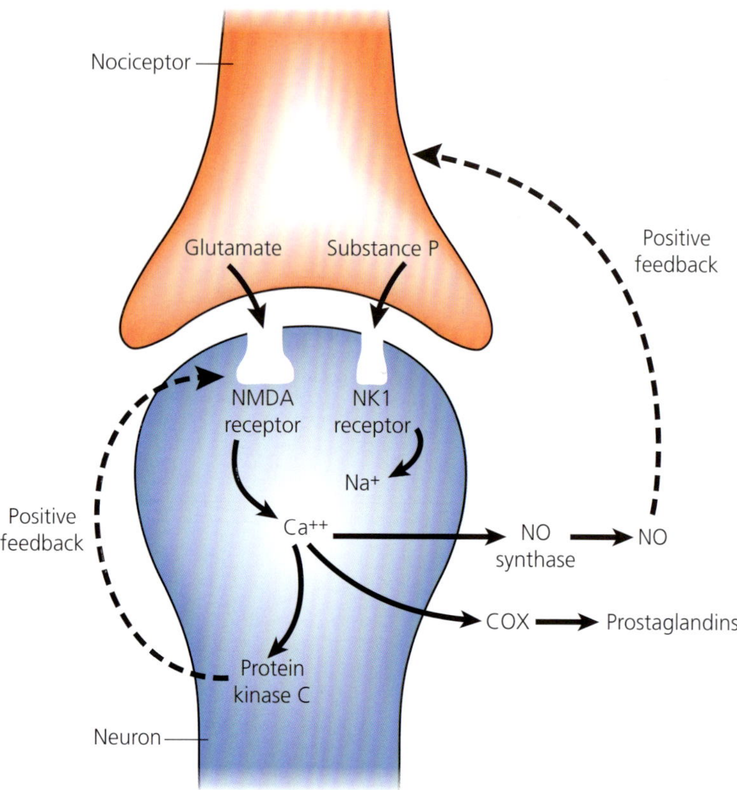

Figure 1.2 Central sensitization/potentiation involves the release of excitatory mediators such as substance P and glutamate by spinal afferent nociceptive neurons in the dorsal horn of the spinal cord. These bind to neurokinin-1 (NK1) and *N*-methyl-D-aspartate (NMDA) receptors, respectively, prompting a massive influx of calcium in the second-order neuron and activating calcium-dependent intracellular enzymes such as protein kinase C, increasing the production of nitric oxide (NO) and prostaglandins. COX, cyclo-oxygenase.

exaggerated responses to afferent impulses and an increased perception of pain (also known as nociplastic pain or pain that arises from altered nociception despite no actual or potential tissue damage).

Clinically, this may present as a progressively exaggerated response to stimuli in an area associated with a specific tissue injury; over time, the sensation encompasses the response to stimuli in the surrounding uninjured tissue as well.

Inhibition. Nociceptive signals also travel through the midbrain and brainstem, where descending inhibitory pathways are activated to dampen pain transmission. These inhibitory pathways are stimulated by endogenous opioids, as well as norepinephrine (noradrenaline) and serotonin; these all modulate the release of inhibitory transmitters such as γ-aminobutyric acid (GABA), glycine, adenosine and additional endogenous opioids at the spinal level. In addition, pain elicits a stress hormone response that promotes the secretion of endogenous opioids from the anterior pituitary and adrenal medulla.

Non-nociceptive pain

Non-nociceptive pain may be divided into neuropathic and psychogenic, with neuropathic pain being further categorized as peripheral or central, depending on the pathogenic mechanism. Psychogenic pain should be considered as a diagnosis of exclusion, when no other nociceptive or neuropathic mechanism can be identified and there are sufficient psychological symptoms to meet the criteria for a somatoform or other defined psychological disorder.

Neuropathic pain is frequently described as burning, tingling, electrical or intense numbness. It may be constant or involve paroxysmal shooting sensations. There are many different types of neuropathic pain that arise from a variety of causes (Table 1.2).

The mechanisms behind neuropathic pain are complex. Injury to a peripheral nerve causes axonal membrane hyperexcitability, leading to spontaneous ectopic impulses that may be perceived as painful. The accumulation of sodium channels at the site of injury lowers the threshold for initiating action potentials. Macrophages migrating to

TABLE 1.2

Types of neuropathic pain and probable causes

Type	Cause
• Trigeminal neuralgia	• Compression of trigeminal ganglion or its branches
• Postherpetic neuralgia	• Shingles (varicella-zoster virus reactivation)
• Complex regional pain syndrome	• Trauma • Infection • Surgery • Inflammation
• Diabetic neuropathy	• Persistent hyperglycemia (diabetes)
• Toxic neuropathy	• Chemotherapy • Radiation therapy
• Central pain	• Trauma to the spinal cord • Stroke
• Phantom pain	• Amputation
• Postincisional pain	• Surgery

the injury site produce inflammatory mediators that contribute to an altered chemical environment surrounding an injured axon, promoting further ectopic activity.

Centrally, nerve injury activates *N*-methyl-D-aspartate (NMDA) and α-amino-3-hydroxy-5-methyl-4-isoxazolepropionic acid (AMPA) receptors, leading to increased intracellular calcium levels and subsequent activation of protein kinase C (PKC) and nitric oxide (NO) synthase (producing NO). Both PKC and

NO enhance neuronal excitability as part of central sensitization (see Figure 1.2).[8]

In addition to the activation of NMDA receptors, upregulation of sodium channels and voltage-sensitive calcium channels in neurons of the dorsal root ganglia may also contribute to spinal cord hyperexcitability (Figure 1.3).

Neuroplasticity. The nervous system is dynamic; it is plastic, in that its structure and function are shaped and reshaped by activity within it, and at each level it continually amplifies or inhibits the signals that the brain ultimately interprets as pain. Appreciating this plasticity is fundamental to the understanding of both the perpetuation of pain in some pain syndromes and the mechanisms of action of pain treatment modalities. There is large variability in the neuroplasticity response among individuals, and this accounts for the large variability in pain response. For example, after surgery

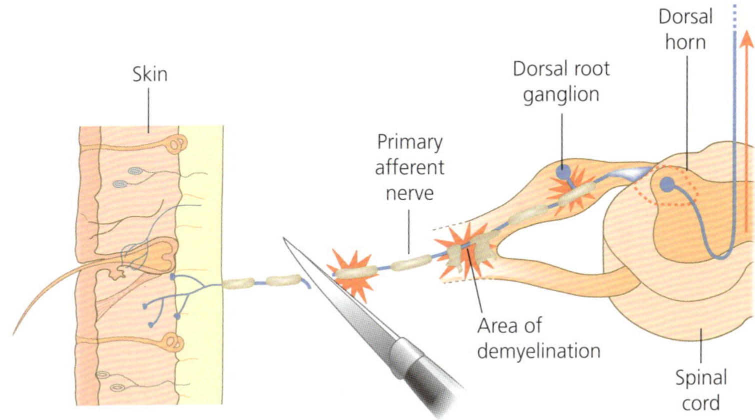

Figure 1.3 Sites of ectopic discharge in damaged peripheral nerves. Hyperactivity occurs at the site of injury, but also near the cell body in the dorsal root ganglion as nerve fibers enter the dorsal horn (area within dashed line). Further ectopic impulses may arise from the demyelinated section of the primary afferent nerve.

or trauma some patients suffer much higher than average acute pain levels. Importantly, these are the people who are at high risk of progression to persistent (chronic) pain (as covered in Chapter 9).[9]

After injury, various growth factors are released, affecting neuronal reorganization as the nerves regenerate (one form of neuroplasticity) (Figure 1.4). Aβ fibers may develop abnormal connections with nociceptive neurons in the dorsal horn, which could contribute to persistent pain hypersensitivity to even non-noxious stimulation.

Non-neuronal cells in the brain and spinal cord called glial cells (microglia) also serve a role in neuronal sensitization and hyperexcitability (Figure 1.5).

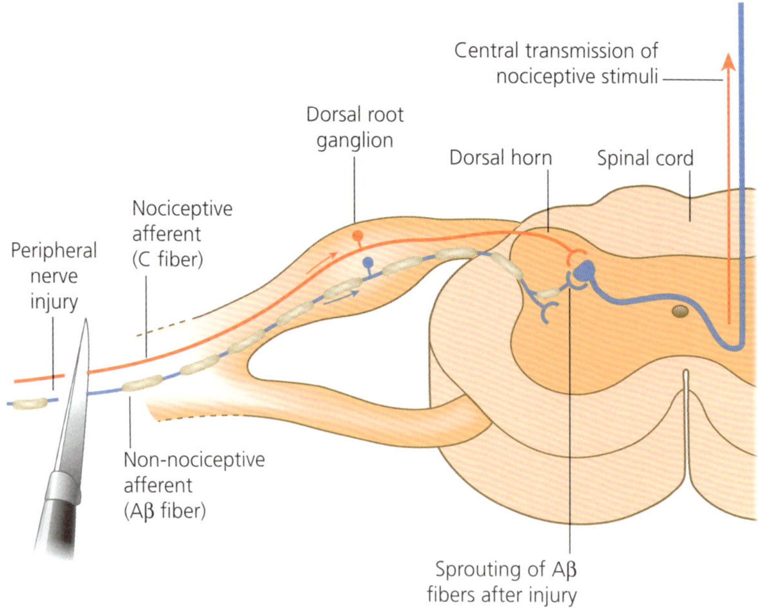

Figure 1.4 Neuronal reorganization. Following peripheral nerve injury, new connections may form between non-nociceptive afferent (Aβ fibers) and nociceptive afferent (C fiber) neurons. These connections contribute to persistent hypersensitivity to pain.

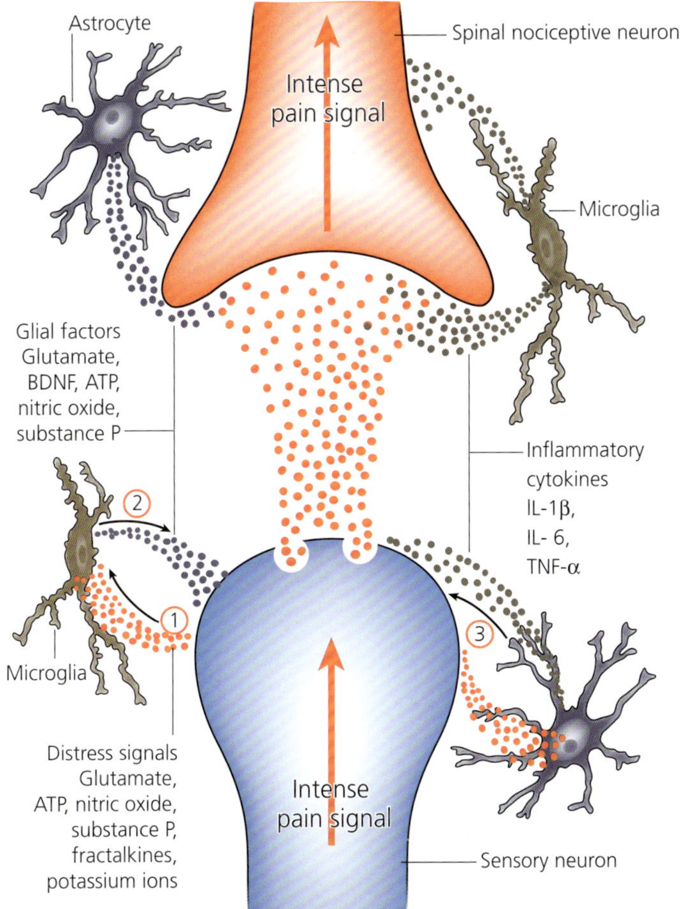

Figure 1.5 (1) After nerve injury, intense signals are transmitted along peripheral sensory neurons to the first synapse in the dorsal horn of the spinal cord. Neurotransmitters cross the synapse to activate spinal neurons. These transmitters are also conveyed to microglia and astrocytes as 'distress signals'. (2) The glial cells produce 'glial factors' and reduce the uptake of neurotransmitters. This either reduces the usual inhibitory processes acting on neurons or stimulates neurons to become hypersensitive. (3) Glial cells are also activated by neural distress signals, which induce the healing process of inflammation through release of inflammatory cytokines, but also result in neuronal sensitization. ATP: adenosine triphosphate; BDNF, brain-derived neurotrophic factor; IL, interleukin; TNF, tumor necrosis factor.

Key points – pain mechanisms

- Pain is an unpleasant sensory and emotional experience associated with actual or potential tissue damage.
- The nervous system is dynamic; not only does it include passive transduction of nociceptive pain signals but also complex processing, resulting in amplification and inhibition of noxious input.
- Nerve injury produces spontaneous ectopic impulses in axons and neurons.
- Understanding the mechanisms involved in the conversion from acute to chronic pain can help identify therapeutic targets.

References

1. International Association for the Study of Pain. IASP terminology. www.iasp-pain.org/Education/Content.aspx?ItemNumber=1698, last accessed 25 June 2020.

2. Bree R. Supplemental guidance on prescribing opioids for postoperative pain. www.breecollaborative.org/wp-content/uploads/Supplemental-Bree-AMDG-Postop-pain-18–0718.pdf, last accessed 25 June 2020.

3. Chou R, Gordon DB, de Leon-Casasola OA et al. Management of postoperative pain: a clinical practice guideline from the American Pain Society, the American Society of Regional Anesthesia and Pain Medicine, and the American Society of Anesthesiologists' Committee on Regional Anesthesia, Executive Committee, and Administrative Council. *J Pain* 2016;17:131–57.

4. Duarte R. Classification of pain. In: Argoff CE, ed. *Pain Management Secrets*, 4th edn. Elsevier, 2018:6–9.

5. Basbaum A. Basic mechanisms. In: Argoff CE, ed. *Pain Management Secrets*, 4th edn. Elsevier, 2018:10–16.

6. Cousins MJ, Gallagher RM. Definitions and mechanisms. In: *Chronic and Cancer Pain*, 2nd edn. Health Press, 2011:7–29.

7. Melzack R, Wall PD. Pain mechanisms: a new theory. *Science* 1965;150:971–9.

8. Apkarian AV, Reckziegel D. Peripheral and central viewpoints of chronic pain, and translational implications. *Neurosci Lett* 2019;702:3–5.

9. Siddall PJ, Cousins MJ. Persistent pain as a disease entity: implications for clinical management. *Anesth Analg* 2004;99:510–20.

2 Preoperative phase

The period leading up to a surgical intervention – or indeed any invasive medical procedure – presents an opportunity to prepare the individual for what they are about to experience and to optimize them from a pain perspective. This chapter discusses the important areas that should be considered and addressed in the preoperative phase to help make the perioperative experience more palatable.

Influencing factors

A large number of disparate factors may influence the development of acute pain. These can be broadly classified into patient, surgical/ anesthetic and institutional/organizational themes.

Patient factors. Acute pain, like any other pain state, is a biopsychosocial construct and therefore the physical and mental state of a patient who is about to undergo a pain-generating procedure can contribute to the nature of the pain experienced. Predictors for the development of more severe acute pain and common themes that transcend the type of surgery undertaken include the following.

- Age: younger age (in an adult surgical population) is an independent predictor of severe postoperative pain.[1,2]
- Psychological morbidity: the presence of preoperative psychological morbidity and distress is a well-documented risk factor. Morbidities include anxiety, depression[3] and insomnia. The somewhat more difficult to define trait of 'pain catastrophizer'[4] is not thought to be linked with risk for acute pain.
- Ethnicity: reporting of pain following a variety of stimuli has been demonstrated to vary between ethnic groups; clinicians should be mindful of this when assessing pain.[5]
- Sex: females have been shown to experience more severe acute pain following surgery,[6,7] though this may be confounded by other risk factors, such as pre-existing pain and age.[8]

- Pre-existing pain in patients undergoing surgery is recognized as a risk factor for the development of severe postoperative pain.[9] This is important as many indications for surgical management, for example arthroplasty, are painful.

Many patients will have a number of risk factors before surgery and some of these may directly influence and modulate each other.[10]

Surgical/anesthetic factors. The type (open versus laparoscopic), duration, urgency and complexity (such as the use of drains or implants) as well as the anatomic site of the surgery can all directly influence the nature of the acute pain experienced. However, the relationship between the surgical insult and the intensity of pain experienced is not as well defined as might first be assumed. In a study of 179 different groups of surgical procedures, some 'minor' procedures such as appendectomy (appendicectomy) and hemorrhoidectomy ranked highly for postoperative pain, possibly because the amount and type of analgesia provided postoperatively were inadequate.[11]

The concept that (perhaps unsurprisingly) the degree of postoperative pain experienced can be heavily influenced by the analgesic regimen adopted is reinforced by a study showing that, for the first day following open and laparoscopic colonic surgery, no difference in pain scores existed between the groups but the open surgery group received more regional anesthetic interventions.[12] Additionally, despite awareness of the importance of delivering adequate analgesia in the perioperative period, it is clear from a number of studies that a high proportion of patients continue to experience moderate to severe pain.[13,14]

The evidence highlights that a 'one-size-fits-all' approach to planning and preparing for perioperative pain management is likely to result in worse outcomes than if a bespoke, personalized approach is taken, factoring in and making provision for the varying influences outlined above.

Institutional/organizational factors. Many aspects of successful perioperative pain management are organizational in nature. Prioritizing effective perioperative pain management may not present a particularly attractive area for administrators and managers to allocate resource to, but it should be emphasized that functional acute pain services deliver cost-effective care.[15,16]

Institutional features. The features of individual institutions are important. Centers with a high-volume throughput of specific surgical interventions are more likely than low-throughput centers to have well-established pathways and protocols for managing these patients during the perioperative period. They are also more likely to have staff who are familiar with the complexities and potential complications that may be encountered in these patient groups. Additionally, those centers that have a high exposure to certain surgeries are more likely to recognize the benefits of investing in relevant equipment, such as patient-controlled analgesia (PCA) pumps, staff training and educational materials for patients.

Identifying those at high risk of severe acute pain allows resources to be targeted to managing these patients effectively in the perioperative period. A robust process of pre-admission screening for risk factors combined with anesthetic pre-assessment allows risk stratification to be undertaken. Regular and effective communication between staff in pre-assessment clinics and clinicians involved in the patient's perioperative journey are of key importance.

Patient education. Time should be taken to educate all patients about what to expect in the perioperative period and to work with them to develop their perioperative pain management plan. This approach is advocated by leading professional bodies.[17,18]

Preoperative assessment

The preoperative phase is important for a number of reasons. First, it enables the patient's current pain status, analgesic consumption and psychological state to be assessed. Second, it provides the opportunity to educate the patient regarding the perioperative period, using the concept of a 'teachable moment',[19] as well as delivering any relevant educational materials that may be available regarding acute postsurgical pain and its management.

Information gathered at the preoperative assessment enables the clinician to assess whether the patient is likely to develop severe acute pain. A patient identified as being high risk should have resources targeted to them – this may manifest as optimization of preoperative analgesia, targeted psychological therapies and/or the development of a personalized pain management plan.

Key points – preoperative phase

- The preoperative phase provides an opportunity to prepare a patient and the team who will be caring for them on the day of surgery.
- Recognized risk factors exist for the development of severe acute postoperative pain – these can be classified as patient, surgical/anesthetic and institutional/organizational factors.
- The preoperative assessment process presents an ideal opportunity to attempt to optimize patients and mitigate risk.

References

1. Kalkman CJ, Visser K, Moen J et al. Preoperative prediction of severe postoperative pain. *Pain* 2003; 105:415–23.

2. Pinto PR, Vieira A, Pereira D, Almeida A. Predictors of acute postsurgical pain after inguinal hernioplasty. *J Pain* 2017;18:947–55.

3. Pan X, Wang J, Lin Z et al. Depression and anxiety are risk factors for postoperative pain-related symptoms and complications in patients undergoing primary total knee arthroplasty in the United States. *J Arthroplasty* 2019;34: 2337–46.

4. Quartana PJ, Campbell CM, Edwards RR. Pain catastrophizing: a critical review. *Expert Rev Neurother* 2009;9:745–58.

5. Campbell CM, Edwards RR. Ethnic differences in pain and pain management. *Pain Manag* 2012; 2:219–30.

6. Gan TJ. Poorly controlled postoperative pain: prevalence, consequences and prevention. *J Pain Res* 2017;10:2287–98.

7. Hah JM, Cramer E, Hilmoe H et al. Factors associated with acute pain estimation, postoperative pain resolution, opioid cessation, and recovery: secondary analysis of a randomized clinical trial. *JAMA Netw Open* 2019;2:e190168.

8. Zheng H, Schnabel A, Yahiaoui-Doktor M et al. Age and preoperative pain are major confounders for sex differences in postoperative pain outcome: a prospective database analysis. *PLoS One* 2017;12:1–14.

9. Erlenwein J, Schlink J, Pfingsten M et al. [Pre-existing pain as comorbidity in postoperative acute pain service.] *Anaesthesist* 2013;62:808–16 [article in German].

10. Ruscheweyh R, Viehoff A, Tio J, Pogatzki-Zahn EM. Psychophysical and psychological predictors of acute pain after breast surgery differ in patients with and without pre-existing chronic pain. *Pain* 2017; 158:1030–8.

11. Gerbershagen HJ, Aduckathil S, van Wijck AJM et al. Pain intensity on the first day after surgery. *Anesthesiology* 2013;118:934–44.

12. Allvin R, Rawal N, Johanzon E, Bäckström R. Open versus laparoscopic surgery: does the surgical technique influence pain outcome? Results from an international registry. *Pain Res Treat* 2016;2016:4087325.

13. Gan TJ, Habib AS, Miller TE et al. Incidence, patient satisfaction, and perceptions of post-surgical pain: results from a US national survey. *Curr Med Res Opin* 2014;30:149–60.

14. Apfelbaum JL, Chen C, Mehta SS, Gan TJ. Postoperative pain experience: results from a national survey suggest postoperative pain continues to be undermanaged. *Anesth Analg* 2003;97:534–40.

15. Lee A, Chan SKC, Chen PP et al. The costs and benefits of extending the role of the acute pain service on clinical outcomes after major elective surgery. *Anesth Analg* 2010;111: 1042–50.

16. Tighe P, Buckenmaier CC, Boezaart AP et al. Acute pain medicine in the United States: a status report. *Pain Med* 2015;16: 1806–26.

17. Chou R, Gordon DB, de Leon-Casasola OA et al. Management of postoperative pain: a clinical practice guideline from the American Pain Society, the American Society of Regional Anesthesia and Pain Medicine, and the American Society of Anesthesiologists' Committee on Regional Anesthesia, Executive Committee, and Administrative Council. *J Pain* 2016;17:131–57.

18. Schug SA, Palmer GM, Scott DA et al. Acute pain management: scientific evidence, fourth edition, 2015. *Med J Aust* 2016;204:315–17.

19. Lawson PJ, Flocke SA. Teachable moments for health behavior change: a concept analysis. *Patient Educ Couns* 2009;76:25–30.

3 Diagnosis and assessment

Pain is a subjective phenomenon, a situation that poses challenges for clinicians when attempting to define, detect and quantify it. Because of pain's somewhat nebulous qualities, the process of assessment is not straightforward and is open to a certain amount of conjecture; common methods of assessing pain are shown in Table 3.1.

What is without doubt is that accurate, regular and reproducible assessment of a patient's pain state in the perioperative period is vitally important. Not only does it guide the administration of analgesic interventions (be they pharmacological or non-pharmacological), it also provides a reliable indication of the clinical trajectory the patient is following after their surgery (acute postsurgical pain should diminish over time), alerting clinicians to potential complications if the expected progress is not made. Finally, attention to the assessment of pain scores and the appropriate actions they trigger is an indicator of a quality healthcare system.

History and physical examination

A comprehensive and accurate history forms the bedrock of pain assessment. In the context of surgery, the intensity of pain is expected to reduce in a progressive fashion from the triggering event (surgical procedure) and its distribution should (generally) relate to the surgical site. Deviation from this pattern can alert the clinician to potential deterioration or the development of surgical complications such as anastomotic leak or infection.[1]

Physical examination can help elucidate the distribution and intensity of pain by direct evaluation of the affected areas or by observation of autonomic responses (sweating, tachycardia, hypertension). From healthcare quality and patient satisfaction perspectives, regular engagement with patients and assessment of their pain enhances their experience and provides reassurance that symptoms are being monitored and recovery supported.

TABLE 3.1

Methods of assessing pain

Method	Benefit	Risk
Physiological parameters (examination)		
• Observation of heart rate, blood pressure, sweatiness	• Easy and cost-effective	• Poor reproducibility
Self-reported assessment tools		
• Often involve a scale	• Simple to use and commonly validated	• Unidimensional • Rely on an individual's understanding of the tool
Observation of behavior		
• Observation and recording of stereotypical behavior believed to represent the presence of pain	• Enables pain to be measured in individuals unable to communicate	• Difficult to administer • Prone to inter-observer variability
Nociception detection devices		
• Measure physical 'markers' of nociception	• May enable nociception to be measured, including in unconscious individuals	• Concerns remain regarding accuracy

Intraoperative assessment of nociception. During surgery, while a patient is under general anesthesia, assessment and quantification of the nociceptive barrage is challenging. An understanding of this parameter is beneficial as it enables intraoperative analgesia to be titrated to effect and potentially enables mitigation of the risk of central sensitization – a process believed to lead to the development of persistent postsurgical pain (see Chapter 9).

A range of non-invasive techniques have been developed to detect and 'quantify' the intraoperative nociception–antinociception (NAN) balance, with a variety of commercial monitors now available. Different approaches have been developed to assess NAN, the majority of which attempt to assess some dimensions of autonomic function. Several of these are detailed below.

The analgesia nociception index (ANI), measured using the PhysioDoloris monitor, provides a surrogate measure of autonomic function by analyzing heart rate variability (HRV). The rationale is that HRV is determined by the supply to the sinoatrial node from the competing sympathetic and parasympathetic nervous systems; higher parasympathetic tone reflects lower levels of nociception. Owing to its reliance on the measurement and interpretation of cardiac parameters, ANI is vulnerable to anything that may interfere with these, such as arrhythmias, pacemakers and antimuscarinic drugs.[2]

The nociception level index. An alternative approach to ANI is to use a broader range of physiological markers. The nociception level (NoL) index, measured by the PMD-200, is a multiparameter composite that combines heart rate, the high-frequency component of HRV, photoplethysmography wave amplitude, skin conductance level and the number and rate of change of skin conductance fluctuations. The index scale ranges from 0 to 100, with higher values indicating greater nociception.

Pupillometers such as the Algiscan and the NeurOptics NPi-200 directly measure the size of a patient's pupils while they undergo surgery. This detects pupil reflex dilation (PRD), which occurs in response to surgical nociceptive stimulation.

Limitations. Although a certain amount of validation work has been undertaken with these devices, they are not widely used. Concerns remain about their accuracy in certain clinical situations, though evidence from studies demonstrates sensitivity and specificity for detecting nociception.[3] As interest in effective perioperative analgesia develops in light of our greater appreciation of aberrant opioid use and the risk poorly controlled acute pain represents for the development of persistent postsurgical pain, it is likely that clinical utilization and research involving these devices will increase.

Detecting and quantifying pain

Many tools have been developed to assist in the measurement of pain intensity and these take a number of forms. For acute pain, the majority of tools are unidimensional and provide a single 'snapshot' of the pain reported. The serial use of these tools and/or assessment of pain during different activity levels ('at rest' and 'on mobilization') is likely to provide more useful clinical information than a single score.

Unidimensional assessment tools are often based on a linear scale, the most commonly encountered being the numerical rating scale ([NRS] 0–10), the visual analog scale (VAS) and the four-point verbal categorical rating scale (Figure 3.1); these provide patients with a means to objectify their pain.[4] There are some criticisms of these tools:

- they lack utility in some patient groups, such as those with learning difficulties or dementia or who are unable to communicate
- patients in pain may find numerical tasks challenging[5]
- a unidimensional tool is unlikely to adequately encompass the complex nature of perioperative pain.

To make unidimensional tools more applicable, a number of specific variations have been developed.

Children. For pediatric patients, a population in which acute pain is commonly encountered, the linear scale has been modified to include visual prompts to help children indicate the level of their pain – an example is the Wong-Baker FACES scale (Figure 3.1).[6] For younger children, observational scales such as the FLACC (face, legs, activity, cry, consolability) scale enable stereotyped behavior to be converted into a pain score.[7]

These scales should be combined with healthcare professionals' understanding and anticipation of potentially painful clinical situations to ensure that acute pain in children is comprehensively assessed and managed.[8]

Patients with dementia or learning difficulties. For elderly people with dementia, another population with a high incidence of pain, or in patients with learning difficulties, self-reporting of pain scores may prove challenging. A more observational approach is required. In patients able to verbalize, providing adequate time to respond and

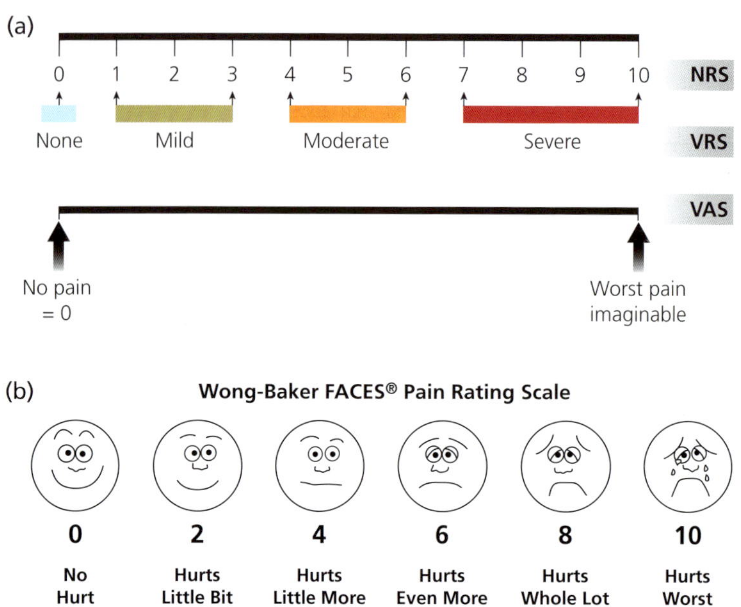

Figure 3.1 Examples of scales used to assess pain. (a) Three unidimensional assessment scales are shown. The NRS relies on a reported number to quantify pain intensity, while the verbal rating scale (VRS) asks patients to describe their level of pain. The VAS requires a patient to indicate their level of pain along a continuum, from no pain to the worst pain imaginable. (b) The self-assessment Wong-Baker FACES® Pain Rating Scale, which is recommended for people aged 3 years and older (not just children). The tool must be understood by the patient, so they are able to choose the face that best illustrates the physical pain they are experiencing. It is not a tool to be used by a third person, parents, healthcare professionals or caregivers, to assess the patient's pain. The Scale is reproduced here with permission from www.WongBakerFACES.org.

using simple descriptor terms often enables the intensity of pain to be effectively communicated.

For non-verbal patients, several scales, including the Abbey, ADD (assessment of discomfort in dementia), CNPI (checklist of nonverbal pain indicator) and Doloplus-2 tools, have been developed and validated for use.[9]

Patients in intensive care present a specific challenge when pain assessment is considered. Although pain is common in this patient population, regular accurate assessment of pain is not. The barriers include the difficulties in communicating with patients who may be delirious, at a low level of consciousness or have airway devices in place.[10] The principle of observation of patient behaviors has been adopted for this cohort. The critical-care pain observation tool (CPOT) combines assessments of facial expression, muscle tension, ventilator compliance (if relevant) and body movements, enabling the assessor to establish the likely level of pain or discomfort experienced.[11]

Digital systems

With the increased use of smart devices and improvements in technology, many commercial companies and healthcare provider systems have developed integrated portals through which patients and healthcare team members can plan the patient's surgical journey, provide information and support through the perioperative period and monitor progress during the postoperative rehabilitative phase. An individual who is not progressing at the expected trajectory can be identified and resource subsequently allocated to support them. This is a rapidly evolving area of clear commercial interest and, as technology advances, new innovations are regularly being developed, deployed and either succeeding or failing. Developments are likely to advance the value of this approach.

Key points – diagnosis and assessment

- Accurate and regular assessment of pain in the perioperative period is vital as it guides the administration of analgesia and provides an indication of the clinical trajectory after surgery.
- Assessment may combine physical examination, observations and the use of validated pain scoring tools. This approach may be tailored to the patient, as necessary.
- Equipment and techniques are being developed to measure intraoperative nociception–antinociception balance.
- Optimal pain assessment serves as a broader indicator of quality care within a healthcare organization.

References

1. Willingham M, Rangrass G, Curcuru C et al. Association between postoperative complications and lingering post-surgical pain: an observational cohort study. *Br J Anaesth* 2020;124:214–21.

2. Ghanty I, Schraag S. The quantification and monitoring of intraoperative nociception levels in thoracic surgery: a review. *J Thorac Dis* 2019;11:4059–71.

3. Funcke S, Sauerlaender S, Pinnschmidt HO et al. Validation of innovative techniques for monitoring nociception during general anesthesia: a clinical study using tetanic and intracutaneous electrical stimulation. *Anesthesiology* 2017; 127:272–83.

4. Breivik H, Borchgrevink PC, Allen SM et al. Assessment of pain. *Br J Anaesth* 2008;101:17–24.

5. Spindler M, Koch K, Borisov E et al. The influence of chronic pain and cognitive function on spatial-numerical processing. *Front Behav Neurosci* 2018;12:1–10.

6. Wong DL, Baker CM. Pain in children: comparison of assessment scales. *Pediatr Nurs* 1988;14:9–17.

7. Merkel SI, Voepel-Lewis T, Shayevitz JR, Malviya S. The FLACC: a behavioral scale for scoring postoperative pain in young children. *Pediatr Nurs* 23:293–7.

8. Hagan J. The assessment and management of acute pain in infants, children, and adolescents. *Pediatrics* 2001;108:793–7.

9. Herr K, Bjoro K, Decker S. Tools for assessment of pain in nonverbal older adults with dementia: a state-of-the-science review. *J Pain Symptom Manage* 2006;31:170–92.

10. Kemp HI, Bantel C, Gordon F et al. Pain Assessment in INTensive care (PAINT): an observational study of physician-documented pain assessment in 45 intensive care units in the United Kingdom. *Anaesthesia* 2017;72:737–48.

11. Gélinas C, Fillion L, Puntillo KA et al. Validation of the critical-care pain observation tool in adult patients. *Am J Crit Care* 2006; 15:420–7.

4 Multimodal strategies

A multimodal approach to postoperative pain care uses a variety of medications, techniques and non-pharmacological strategies to target different areas within the central and/or peripheral nervous system (Table 4.1 and Figure 4.1). Such an approach provides superior analgesia to that obtained using one agent.[1] Consequently, multimodal analgesia can reduce opioid consumption and the associated side effects while supporting improved functional status during postoperative recovery.[2,3]

A well-balanced pain plan should not be limited to systemic pharmacological therapies. It may involve neuraxial and peripheral regional anesthetic techniques, local and/or topical pharmacological therapies, physical modalities such as ice and heat, and cognitive–behavioral modalities.

Regimen selection

When choosing a multimodal regimen, it is important to invoke a broad spectrum of treatment modalities while also keeping in mind the side effects and safety profile of each agent.

In general, using agents across different categories of multimodal analgesia is recommended. Based on the available studies, some components have strong support for use in specific surgical procedures, while there is a paucity of evidence for others.

Systemic pharmacotherapies

Opioids, paracetamol (acetaminophen) and non-steroidal anti-inflammatory drugs (NSAIDs) are ubiquitously recommended for postoperative pain management. Gabapentin or pregabalin are also frequently incorporated into multimodal regimens, depending on the surgery type and patient risk factors.[4]

Paracetamol/NSAIDs. One of the simplest options is to include, when possible, scheduled paracetamol and/or NSAIDs; these tend to be well

TABLE 4.1

Components of a multimodal approach

Systemic pharmacological

- Opioids
- NSAIDs
- Paracetamol (acetaminophen)
- Anticonvulsants (gabapentin/pregabalin)
- IV ketamine infusion
- IV lidocaine infusion
- IV magnesium
- α_2-agonists (clonidine/dexmedetomidine)

Non-pharmacological cognitive

- Guided imagery
- Relaxation
- Hypnosis
- Distraction
- Music therapy
- Virtual reality
- Intraoperative suggestion

Procedural

- Local anesthetic infiltration at incision
- Intra-articular local anesthetic
- Site-specific regional anesthesia block with local anesthetic
- Epidural with local anesthetic ± opioid
- Intrathecal opioid

Local/topical pharmacological

- Menthol cream
- Topical local anesthetic (cream or patch)
- Topical NSAID
- Capsaicin cream

Non-pharmacological physical

- Transcutaneous electrical nerve stimulation (TENS)
- Ice/heat
- Acupuncture
- Massage
- Continuous passive motion

IV, intravenous.

tolerated, with most studies indicating less postoperative pain and reduced opioid consumption when either one is used in combination with opioid compared with opioid alone.[5,6]

Patient risk factors such as liver dysfunction and history of significant alcohol use will need to be accounted for when using paracetamol, just as renal function, history of gastric ulcer or history of cardiovascular disease will affect the safety of NSAIDs.

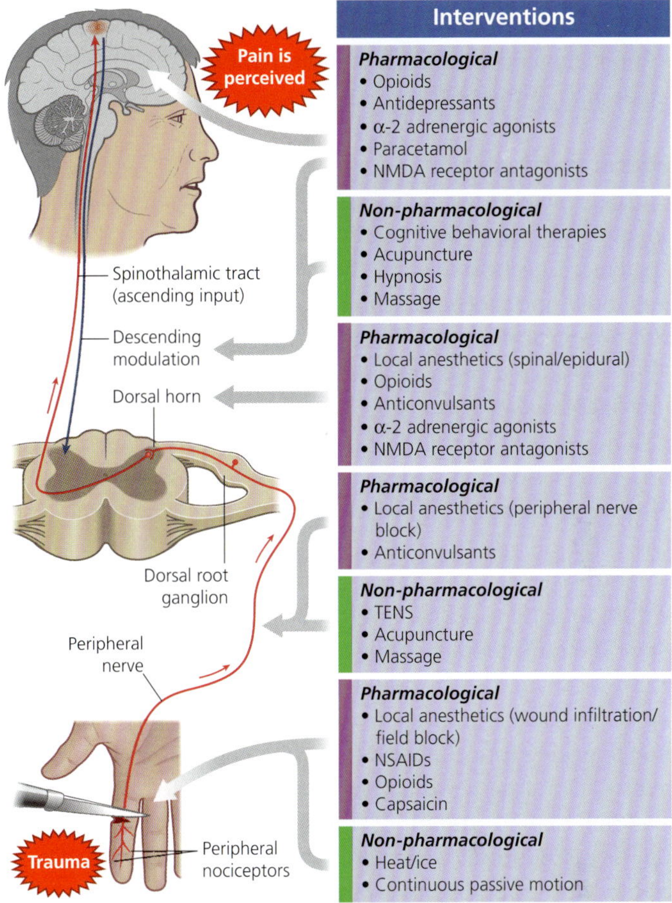

Figure 4.1 Targets of multimodal therapies. Each analgesic agent may work on one or multiple sites throughout the nervous system to interfere with each phase of the nociceptive pathway while also attenuating processes leading to central sensitization. The figure does not include all possible interventions, but it represents a large selection with the predominant mechanisms of action indicated. Systemic medications such as opioids and NMDA receptor antagonists (ketamine) have important roles in perception and descending inhibitory pathways, whereas local anesthetics administered epidurally and anticonvulsants will have greater effect on transmission through the nervous system. Meanwhile, NSAIDs and topical agents will reduce transduction at a local level. TENS, transcutaneous electrical nerve stimulation.

Intravenous ketamine and lidocaine are strongly supported for major surgical procedures, with predominant evidence for lidocaine in intra-abdominal surgery.

Procedural techniques

Appropriately targeted regimens are beneficial in various specific surgeries. Although the choice of peripheral nerve block, neuraxial analgesia or intra-articular injection may not be clearly guided by evidence, generally only one procedure should be employed at a given time.

As for non-pharmacological treatments, cognitive modalities should be considered given generally positive results in studies and the very low likelihood of harm (see Chapter 7). Using transcutaneous electrical nerve stimulation (TENS) as an adjunct has evidence-based support, while modalities such as acupuncture, massage or cold therapy need further study. Again, however, the risks are low with these options.

Minimizing risk

In addition to patient risk factors, the selection of therapies for inclusion in a multimodal regimen should not create undue risks. Generally, local anesthesia should be administered only through one route to avoid local anesthesia toxicity. For example, combining a systemic lidocaine infusion with a peripheral nerve catheter infusing another local anesthetic would not be recommended. On the other hand, adding a small amount of topical local anesthetic to an area outside the distribution of the peripheral nerve catheter may be reasonable, with careful consideration.

Similarly, caution should be used when administering opioids through more than one route. If a patient has patient-controlled epidural anesthesia (PCEA) with local anesthesia and opioid infusing, additional externally administered oral or parenteral opioids may not be appropriate.

Timing

The best time to initiate multimodal analgesia is not clear. Patient education in cognitive techniques such as guided imagery and relaxation may be more appropriately accomplished preoperatively, to allow patients to use these methods throughout the immediate perioperative period.

Pre-emptive analgesia may offer some advantages, as has been demonstrated with epidural analgesia and local anesthetic wound infiltration.[7] Multiple studies have also revealed benefit from preoperative analgesia with agents such as gabapentin, paracetamol and NSAIDs (for example, celecoxib).[8] The ideal dosing, timing and duration of continued systemic therapy are unclear for each adjunct. It is believed that round-the-clock dosing of non-opioid adjuncts reduces or may even eliminate the need for opioid analgesics in some patients.

The intraoperative period is also a key time to use multimodal analgesia. The concept of opioid-free anesthesia is long established; commonly used agents include intravenous (IV) lidocaine, ketamine, dexmedetomidine and magnesium infusions (which may include boluses of medication prior to initiation of a lower-dose infusion).

Opioid-free anesthesia can successfully be performed with adequate pain control and excellent postoperative recovery, even without utilization of regional or neuraxial blockade, which highlights how effective different systemic pharmacological approaches can be when used in combination.[9]

Key points – multimodal strategies

- Multimodal analgesia uses a variety of medications, techniques and non-pharmacological options to target different areas of the central and/or peripheral nervous system for a synergistic effect.
- Multimodal analgesia improves the quality of pain treatment while reducing opioid use and its associated side effects.
- When choosing specific treatment options, side effects and safety profiles should be considered.
- Components of multimodal analgesia can be implemented preoperatively, intraoperatively and postoperatively.

References

1. Schwenk ES, Mariano ER. Designing the ideal perioperative pain management plan starts with multimodal analgesia. *Korean J Anesthesiol* 2018;71:345–52.

2. Kehlet H, Dahl JB. The value of 'multimodal' or 'balanced analgesia' in postoperative pain treatment. *Anesth Analg* 1993;77:1048–56.

3. Basse L, Jakobsen DH, Bardram L et al. Functional recovery after open versus laparoscopic colonic resection: a randomized, blinded study. *Ann Surg* 2005;241:416–23.

4. Tiippana EM, Hamunen K, Kontinen VK, Kalso E. Do surgical patients benefit from perioperative gabapentin/pregabalin? A systematic review of efficacy and safety. *Anesth Analg* 2007;104:1545–56.

5. Maund E, McDaid C, Rice S et al. Paracetamol and selective and non-selective non-steroidal anti-inflammatory drugs for the reduction in morphine-related side-effects after major surgery: a systematic review. *Br J Anaesth* 2011;106:292–7.

6. Elia N, Lysakowski C, Tramèr MR. Does multimodal analgesia with acetaminophen, nonsteroidal antiinflammatory drugs, or selective cyclooxygenase-2 inhibitors and patient-controlled analgesia morphine offer advantages over morphine alone? Meta-analyses of randomized trials. *Anesthesiology* 2005;103:1296–304.

7. Gottschalk A, Smith DS. New concepts in acute pain therapy: preemptive analgesia. *Am Fam Physician* 2001;63:1979–84.

8. Ong CK, Lirk P, Seymour RA, Jenkins BJ. The efficacy of preemptive analgesia for acute postoperative pain management: a meta-analysis. *Anesth Analg* 2005;100:757–73.

9. Mauermann E, Ruppen W, Bandschapp O. Different protocols used today to achieve total opioid-free general anesthesia without locoregional blocks. *Best Pract Res Clin Anaesthesiol* 2017;31:533–45.

5 Systemic therapies

Systemic pharmacological agents are the most commonly used therapies for acute pain treatment, particularly when more than one region of the body is affected. NSAIDs and/or paracetamol should be considered first-line therapy for all acute pain treatment (assuming no contraindications) and may be sufficient for some minor procedures, such as dental surgery.[1]

For more severe pain, opioids and gabapentinoids can be considered, in addition. For inpatients, ketamine, lidocaine, magnesium and dexmedetomidine infusions may be options for complex or severe pain.

The aim of using multiple different systemic agents is not just to improve pain care, but also to reduce opioid use and avoid harmful side effects (see Chapter 4).[2,3]

NSAIDs and paracetamol

NSAIDs have been used for centuries, yet their mechanism of action was only linked to the inhibition of prostaglandin synthesis in 1971.[4] Although the existence of cyclo-oxygenase (COX) isoenzymes had been postulated, it was not until 1989 that a second distinct protein with COX activity was isolated.[5]

The identification of a constitutively expressed enzyme in almost all human tissues (COX-1) and an alternative, highly regulated, enzyme predominantly expressed in states of inflammation (COX-2) resulted in the theory that COX-1 inhibition was responsible for many of the side effects associated with NSAIDs (Figure 5.1).[6] The development of COX-2-specific inhibitors, and the prospect of anti-inflammatory effects with fewer adverse effects,[7,8] was welcomed enthusiastically by clinicians and patients alike. The popularity of these novel agents increased rapidly. However, many were subsequently withdrawn from the market because of associations with excess relative risks of cardiovascular and cerebrovascular events.[9]

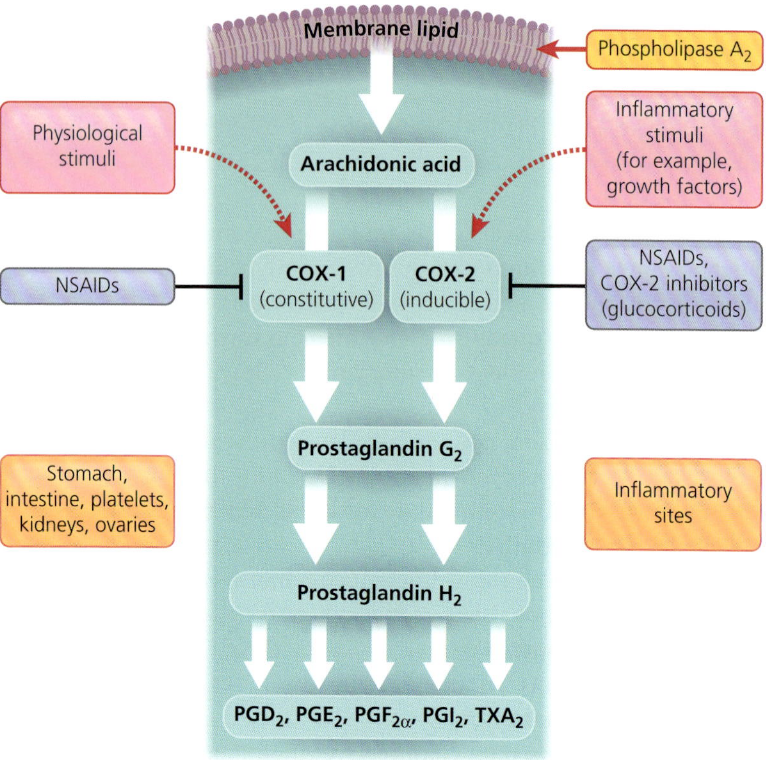

Figure 5.1 The arachidonic acid cascade. Arachidonic acid, which is a normal component of membrane phospholipid, is released by phospholipase A_2. COX-1 and COX-2 metabolize it to prostaglandins G_2 and H_2, which are further converted to other prostaglandins (PGs) and thromboxane A_2 (TXA_2).

Potential risks. A number of systematic reviews have explored the added risk NSAIDs pose to surgical patients. They have been postulated to influence the development of complications, including wound infection, anastomotic leak, kidney injury, delayed bone healing and hemorrhage.

In oncology patients undergoing gut resection, there was no conclusive evidence that the use of NSAIDs in the perioperative period led to an increased risk of anastomotic leak or recurrence.[10]

By inhibiting COX and platelet thromboxane A_2, NSAIDs reduce platelet aggregation and vasoconstriction, leading to impaired coagulation and prolonged bleeding time. In a systematic review that included more than 1700 patients receiving plastic surgery, the risk of bleeding complications in patients who had used NSAIDs was twice that of those who had not (though the risk was still low),[11] a situation mirrored in joint surgery[12] and Roux-en-Y gastric bypass surgery.[13]

Conversely, in tonsillectomy NSAIDs do not appear to increase the risk of postoperative bleeding.[14]

Postoperative hemorrhage often has multiple contributory factors and the most prudent approach is to avoid this class of drugs in patients with increased bleeding risk or during/after surgery where bleeding has been an issue.

The development of wound infections, a scenario in which host inflammation provides a degree of innate protection, has been suggested to be adversely influenced by the use of NSAIDs. In an animal model of *Streptococcus pyogenes* wound infection, ibuprofen increased the risk of tissue necrosis and more severe infection,[15] while in another animal model, diclofenac had no effect on wound healing.[16] In general, the evidence of an increased risk of wound infection or breakdown in humans remains inconclusive.[17]

Principles of use. As with all interventions suggested in this book, a personalized approach based on risk versus benefit should be adopted when using NSAIDs in the perioperative period. The demographics and medical history of the patient and the nature of surgery should be considered. To minimize the risk of side effects, the guiding principles can be summarized as: use the lowest possible dose of NSAID for the shortest period of time.[18] Gastroprotective strategies are also advised – use a proton pump inhibitor for patients judged to be at risk of NSAID-mediated gut damage.

Examples of NSAIDs and dosing strategies are shown in Table 5.1.

Paracetamol has a mechanism of action that is not completely understood. It seems to inhibit COX activity in the brain but, unlike NSAIDs, it does not inhibit function outside the nervous system and is therefore not useful as an anti-inflammatory.

Paracetamol, when used with other analgesic agents, reduces postoperative opioid use. It may be administered by mouth or intravenously – neither route is considered superior. The primary limitation is the potential for liver toxicity. The dose should be limited

TABLE 5.1

Sample dosing strategies for NSAIDs and paracetamol

Drug	Dose	Comments
Ibuprofen	Oral: 400–800 mg, 3–4 times daily	• All NSAIDs may cause GI bleeding and ulceration, renal dysfunction and cardiac events with prolonged use • Contraindicated after CABG
Ketorolac	IV: 7.5–15 mg, 3–4 times daily	• Limit to 5 days
Celecoxib	Oral: 400 mg daily or 50–200 mg twice a day	• Reduced risk of bleeding with COX-2 inhibitors such as celecoxib
Paracetamol	Oral/IV: 500–1000 mg every 6 hours, to maximum 4 g/day	• Reduce maximum dose to 3 g in elderly • Reduce maximum dose to 2 g with hepatic dysfunction • May cause hepatotoxicity

CABG, coronary artery bypass grafting; GI, gastrointestinal.

to 4 g in 24 hours in adults, with a reduction to 2 g in 24 hours for patients with significant alcohol use or history of hepatitis C and to 3 g in 24 hours in elderly individuals.

Opioids

Opioid medications are very effective for moderate to severe acute pain. Their effect is generally attributed to binding at three principal opioid receptors: μ, κ and δ. These G-protein-coupled receptors modulate calcium and potassium entry into neuronal membranes, causing hyperpolarization of nociceptive cell membranes (Figure 5.2). In turn, this shortens the duration of action potentials and inhibits the release of excitatory mediators, producing analgesia.

Side effects. Opioids are, unfortunately, associated with a slew of side effects, ranging from nausea, vomiting, constipation and pruritus to urinary retention, altered mental status and drowsiness. Perhaps the

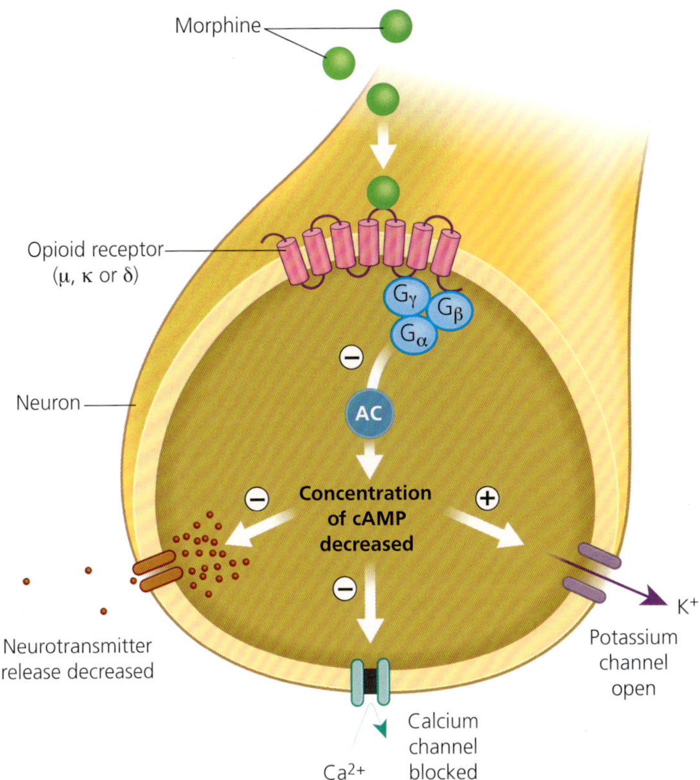

Figure 5.2 Mechanism of action of an opioid. Binding at the opioid receptor, which is G-protein coupled, inhibits adenylate cyclase (AC), decreasing the intracellular concentration of cyclic AMP (cAMP), which in turn inhibits calcium influx and increases potassium efflux.

most concerning side effect is respiratory depression, which can lead to brain injury and death. Particular care should be taken to monitor for respiratory effects in patients with risk factors such as chronic obstructive pulmonary disease (COPD) and obstructive sleep apnea and efforts should be made to minimize other sedating medications, such as benzodiazepines, which may significantly increase the risk of harmful respiratory events.

Patients develop tolerance to the adverse effects of opioids over time, with the exception of constipation. A prophylactic bowel regimen should be initiated, including a stool softener and/or stimulant agent.

Principles of use. The lowest effective dose of opioid should be used, with escalation based on functional gains and side effects. Opioids come in many different formulations, and they may be administered via oral, IV, transdermal, intrathecal/epidural and sublingual/transmucosal routes (Table 5.2).

In patients able to tolerate it, the oral route is preferred over IV administration as the analgesic effects are similar. Because of safety concerns and the inability to titrate the dose easily, long-acting oral opioids are not recommended for use in the immediate postoperative period other than for patients already using them long term.

When the parenteral route is required, PCA should be considered. Basal infusions should not be used in opioid-naive adults, as they are associated with an increased risk of side effects without improved analgesia.

TABLE 5.2

Commonly used opioid medications in periprocedural pain treatment

Route	Medication
Oral	• Oxycodone • Hydromorphone • Morphine • Hydrocodone • Tramadol
IV	• Hydromorphone • Morphine • Fentanyl • Nalbuphine
Other	• Fentanyl lozenge • Buprenorphine sublingual

Choice of medication should be based on potency as well as desired duration of action and side-effect profile. For example, morphine should be avoided in patients with renal failure. Further, IV fentanyl or fentanyl lozenges may be useful during shorter, defined pain events such as wound care.

Intramuscular administration should be discouraged because of unreliable absorption.

Clear efforts are being made worldwide to reduce use of opioids when reasonable. Concerns have been raised – particularly in the USA and Canada – regarding overprescribing for both acute and chronic pain leading to the potential for new addiction, overdose or diversion.[19] Regardless of the opioid epidemic, however, there are advantages to using opioid-sparing techniques to reduce side effects.

Anticonvulsants

The anticonvulsants gabapentin and pregabalin are commonly used perioperatively. They bind voltage-gated calcium channels to inhibit the release of excitatory neurotransmitters. Although these medications were initially studied in chronic neuropathic pain, they have also been shown to reduce acute pain and opioid use in acute pain settings.[20,21]

Doses and regimens vary widely. Many trials have evaluated gabapentin at doses of 600–1200 mg, three times daily, or pregabalin at 150–300 mg/day preoperatively, with possible continuation of the medication afterwards (Table 5.3). The dose should be reduced with renal dysfunction, though the medications themselves are not nephrotoxic. Dose reductions are also appropriate in older patients and where sedation is a concern. For patients predisposed to seizures, anticonvulsants should be tapered over 1 week rather than abruptly discontinued.

Side effects include sedation, peripheral edema, dizziness and tremor.

Magnesium infusions intraoperatively and postoperatively have also been associated with decreased postoperative pain and reduced nausea and vomiting. Magnesium is not a primary analgesic, but it may enhance the role of other analgesics through its blockade of the NMDA receptor and calcium channels and blunting of somatic and autonomic responses to noxious stimuli.

Doses are commonly a bolus of 30–50 mg/kg followed by a maintenance dose of 6–20 mg/kg/hour (Table 5.3). Magnesium can potentiate the effects of non-depolarizing muscle relaxants used intraoperatively, and anesthesiologists may need to adjust doses accordingly.

TABLE 5.3

Sample dosing strategies for anticonvulsants

Drug	Dose	Comments
Gabapentin	Oral: 600–1200 mg three times a day	• Can cause dizziness, sedation, peripheral edema • Reduce dose in renal failure
Pregabalin	Oral: 150–300 mg/day in 2–3 divided doses	• Greater bioavailability than gabapentin
Magnesium	IV bolus: 30–50 mg/kg Infusion: 6–20 mg/kg/hour	• Interacts with non-depolarizing muscle relaxants

Ketamine

Ketamine is a dissociative anesthetic that has hypnotic, analgesic and amnestic effects. At subanesthetic doses, it has roles in acute and chronic pain, and it is associated with decreased postoperative pain scores and decreased risk of persistent postsurgical pain.[22]

Ketamine works by inhibiting NMDA-gated calcium channels. It has been shown to be particularly helpful in the treatment of pain in opioid-tolerant patients and to reduce pain for weeks to months after surgery in patients with chronic pain. It should also be considered for opioid-naive patients, as part of a multimodal treatment strategy.

Dosing regimens of ketamine vary according to, among other variables, whether use is pre-, intra- or postoperative. Analgesic dose ranges are wide, with boluses of 0.3–0.5 mg/kg and infusions ranging from 0.1 mg/kg/hour to 0.2 mg/kg/hour (Table 5.4). Higher doses are more likely to be associated with side effects.

Side effects. The most common side effects of ketamine include hallucinations, nightmares, nystagmus and increased salivation. Caution should be used in patients with significant psychiatric comorbidities, including history of psychosis, mania and

TABLE 5.4

Sample dosing strategy for ketamine (NMDA antagonist)

Dose	Comments
IV bolus: 0.3–0.5 mg/kg Infusion: 0.1–0.2 mg/kg/hour	• Avoid in patients with history of psychosis • May cause hallucinations, nightmares, dysphoria, nystagmus, excessive salivation

post-traumatic stress disorder (PTSD). Increased intracranial pressure and increased sympathetic activity are more likely to occur at higher doses. Consequently, ketamine should be avoided in individuals with intracranial pathology or significant coronary artery disease.

Lidocaine

Lidocaine can be delivered via IV infusion, peripheral nerve block, neuraxial techniques and topical formulations (discussed predominantly in Chapter 6). Lidocaine infusions have analgesic advantages beyond the classic blocking of nociceptive transmission associated with local anesthetics.[23]

Systemic lidocaine has analgesic, antihyperalgesic and anti-inflammatory properties. It has been shown to promote an earlier return of bowel function after open abdominal procedures. Although opioid sparing, the effect size may not be as great as with an epidural in abdominal procedures.[24] However, it remains an excellent option for patients with contraindications to neuraxial or regional approaches (such as anticoagulation concern). If a patient is receiving a lidocaine infusion, administration of local anesthetics through another route, such as peripheral nerve block, should be avoided to reduce the risk of local anesthetic toxicity.

Dosing. Intravenous lidocaine dosing is weight based. Generally, lidocaine is delivered as a continuous infusion of 1–2 mg/kg/hour, which may or may not be preceded by a bolus of 1.5 mg/kg (Table 5.5). It may be used intraoperatively and continued for 24–48 hours postoperatively.

TABLE 5.5

Sample dosing strategy for lidocaine (local anesthetic)

Dose	Comment
IV bolus: 1.5 mg/kg Infusion: 1–2 mg/kg/hour	• Can cause dizziness, seizures, cardiac arrhythmias, bradycardia

Side effects include dizziness, tinnitus, perioral numbness, seizures, conduction block and bradycardia. Absolute contraindications include first- and second-degree heart block. Relative contraindications include concomitant use of β-blockers or α-agonists. Caution should be used in patients with underlying liver dysfunction – elimination may be reduced, predisposing the patient to local anesthetic toxicity.

α-2 agonists

α-2 agonists such as dexmedetomidine and clonidine are commonly used as adjuncts to reduce opioid consumption, postoperative nausea and vomiting and intraoperative stress responses.[25] The medications stimulate α-2 adrenergic receptors in the central nervous system, causing hyperpolarization of neurons by reducing potassium efflux and increasing calcium influx. This hyperpolarization reduces norepinephrine release as well as inhibiting nociceptive neuronal firing. Table 5.6 shows sample dosing strategies for dexmedetomidine and clonidine.

Dexmedetomidine has a much higher affinity for α-2 receptors when compared with clonidine. It may cause bradycardia and hypotension with ongoing use and severe hypertension with a loading dose. It is most commonly used intraoperatively or in an intensive care setting.

Clonidine is also associated with hypotension, but it may cause severe hypertension if stopped abruptly.

TABLE 5.6

Sample dosing strategies for α-2 agonists

Drug	Dose	Comments
Dexmedetomidine	IV bolus: 0.5–1 µg/kg over 10 mins Infusion: 0.2–1.7 µg/kg/hour	• Loading dose may cause hypertension • Can cause severe bradycardia and hypotension
Clonidine	Oral: 0.2 mg twice a day	• Can cause severe hypotension • May cause hypertension when stopped

Key points – systemic therapies

- NSAIDs and/or paracetamol should be considered first-line therapy for all acute pain treatment (assuming no contraindications); they may be sufficient for some minor procedures.
- Opioids are effective for treating acute postprocedural pain, but use should be minimized to reduce side effects, which may include respiratory depression, drowsiness, nausea, vomiting, constipation, pruritus and urinary retention. Care should be taken to use the lowest effective dose.
- Gabapentin and pregabalin can be useful oral adjuncts, initiated preoperatively and continued through postoperative recovery, for select patients and procedures.
- Several IV agents, including ketamine, lidocaine, dexmedetomidine and magnesium, are useful as part of a multimodal opioid-sparing approach that can be used intraoperatively and/or postoperatively.

References

1. Ong CK, Seymour RA, Lirk P, Merry AF. Combining paracetamol (acetaminophen) with nonsteroidal antiinflammatory drugs: a qualitative systematic review of analgesic efficacy for acute postoperative pain. *Anesth Analg* 2010;110:1170–9.

2. Wick EC, Grant MC, Wu CL. Postoperative multimodal analgesia pain management with nonopioid analgesics and techniques: a review. *JAMA Surg* 2017;152:691–7.

3. Chou R, Gordon DB, de Leon-Casasola OA et al. Management of postoperative pain: a clinical practice guideline from the American Pain Society, the American Society of Regional Anesthesia and Pain Medicine, and the American Society of Anesthesiologists' Committee on Regional Anesthesia, Executive Committee, and Administrative Council. *J Pain* 2016;17:131–57.

4. Vane JR. Inhibition of prostaglandin synthesis as a mechanism of action for aspirin-like drugs. *Nat New Biol* 1971;231:237–9.

5. Rosen GD, Birkenmeier TM, Raz A, Holtzman MJ. Identification of a cyclooxygenase-related gene and its potential role in prostaglandin formation. *Biochem Biophys Res Commun* 1989;164:1358–65.

6. Cashman JN. The mechanisms of action of NSAIDs in analgesia. *Drugs* 1996;52:13–23.

7. Bombardier C, Laine L, Reicin A et al. Comparison of upper gastrointestinal toxicity of rofecoxib and naproxen in patients with rheumatoid arthritis. *N Engl J Med* 2000;343:1520–8.

8. Silverstein FE, Faich G, Goldstein JL et al. Gastrointestinal toxicity with celecoxib vs nonsteroidal anti-inflammatory drugs for osteoarthritis and rheumatoid arthritis. *JAMA* 2000;284:1247–55.

9. Halpern GM. COX-2 inhibitors: a story of greed, deception and death. *Inflammopharmacology* 2005; 13:419–25.

10. Cata JP, Guerra CE, Chang GJ et al. Non-steroidal anti-inflammatory drugs in the oncological surgical population: beneficial or harmful? A systematic review of the literature. *Br J Anaesth* 2017;119:750–64.

11. Forsyth MG, Clarkson DJ, O'Boyle CP. A systematic review of the risk of postoperative bleeding with perioperative non-steroidal anti-inflammatory drugs (NSAIDs) in plastic surgery. *Eur J Plast Surg* 2018;41:505–10.

12. Schafer AI. Effects of nonsteroidal anti-inflammatory therapy on platelets. *Am J Med* 1999;106:25S–36S.

13. Klein M, Stockei M, Rosenberg J, Gögenur I. Intraoperative ketorolac and bleeding after laparoscopic Roux-en-Y gastric by-pass surgery. *Acta Chir Belg* 2012;112:369–73.

14. Krishna S, Hughes LF, Lin SY. Postoperative hemorrhage with nonsteroidal anti-inflammatory drug use after tonsillectomy: a meta-analysis. *Arch Otolaryngol Head Neck Surg* 2003;129:1086–9.

15. Weng TC, Chen CC, Toh HS, Tang HJ. Ibuprofen worsens *Streptococcus pyogenes* soft tissue infections in mice. *J Microbiol Immunol Infect* 2011;44:418–23.

16. Klein M, Krarup P-M, Kongsbak MB et al. Effect of postoperative diclofenac on anastomotic healing, skin wounds and subcutaneous collagen accumulation: a randomized, blinded, placebo-controlled, experimental study. *Eur Surg Res* 2012;48:73–8.

17. Zhao-Fleming H, Hand A, Zhang K et al. Effect of non-steroidal anti-inflammatory drugs on postsurgical complications against the backdrop of the opioid crisis. *Burn Trauma* 2018;6:1–9.

18. National Institute for Health and Care Excellence. Non-steroidal anti-inflammatory drugs: KTT13. London: NICE, 2015, last updated 2018. www.nice.org.uk/advice/ktt13, last accessed 14 July 2020.

19. Koepke EJ, Manning EL, Miller TE et al. The rising tide of opioid use and abuse: the role of the anesthesiologist. *Perioper Med (Lond)* 2018;7:16.

20. Clarke H, Bonin RP, Orser BA et al. The prevention of chronic postsurgical pain using gabapentin and pregabalin: a combined systematic review and meta-analysis. *Anesth Analg* 2012;115:428–42.

21. Verret M, Lauzier F, Zarychanski R et al. Perioperative use of gabapentinoids for the management of postoperative acute pain: protocol of a systematic review and meta-analysis. *Syst Rev* 2019;8:24.

22. Schwenk ES, Viscusi ER, Buvanendran A et al. Consensus guidelines on the use of intravenous ketamine infusions for acute pain management from the American Society of Regional Anesthesia and Pain Medicine, the American Academy of Pain Medicine, and the American Society of Anesthesiologists. *Reg Anesth Pain Med* 2018;43:456–66.

23. Weibel S, Jelting Y, Pace NL et al. Continuous intravenous perioperative lidocaine infusion for postoperative pain and recovery in adults. *Cochrane Database Syst Rev* 2018;6:CD009642.

24. Eipe N, Gupta S, Penning J. Intravenous lidocaine for acute pain: an evidence-based clinical update. *BJA Education* 2016;16:292–8.

25. Blaudszun G, Lysakowski C, Elia N, Tramèr MR. Effect of perioperative systemic α2 agonists on postoperative morphine consumption and pain intensity: systematic review and meta-analysis of randomized controlled trials. *Anesthesiology* 2012;116:1312–22.

6 Non-systemic therapies

Local anesthetic drugs, administered neuraxially, perineurally or as a surgical 'field block', have played a role in the perioperative management of pain for over a century. Techniques have developed hand in hand with advances in pharmacology, imaging techniques and the equipment used to deliver the relevant drugs to the appropriate anatomic site. Interest in these non-systemic approaches has grown as a truly multimodal approach to controlling perioperative pain is increasingly advocated and adopted. This chapter presents the relevant features of the non-systemic methods that can be adopted and strategies for integrating them into the perioperative analgesic regimen.

General principles and considerations

Local anesthetic agents block the transmission of action potentials along nerves in a 'use-dependent' fashion. Administration of local anesthetic in close proximity to nerve tissue renders the nerves unable to function. In the case of sensory neurons, this renders insensate the area innervated by these nerves.

The duration of action of local anesthetic agents varies. Their effective half-life is influenced by both the metabolism of the drug and the rate of elimination by the vasculature from the tissues where it is intended to have an effect (a process that can be slowed by co-administration with a vasoconstrictor).[1] At its most basic level, the injection or infiltration of local anesthetic into the tissues which comprise the area of surgery, commonly termed a 'surgical field block', will result in a reduction in nociception at the time of the surgical insult and, depending on the agent used, for a period of time after.

Catheter use. Prolonging the duration of effect of a variety of blocks can be achieved by infusing local anesthetic along catheters placed:

- centrally, for example, in the epidural space

- peripherally along major nerves, such as the femoral nerve
- in anatomic spaces or planes traversed by nerves, such as the paravertebral space or transverse abdominis plane.

The benefits of using a catheter-based approach to delivery relate to the duration and density of the block that can be achieved, which is often of such quality that little additional analgesia may be required.

The potential downsides are relatively numerous and include risks during catheter insertion (damage to anatomic structures), risks of overdose and toxicity and wrong-route administration errors. The occurrence of these events can be reduced by comprehensive training and support of staff.

Improving safety. Advanced techniques are needed for the administration of many blocks, and clinicians who undertake them should have adequate training and experience. Additionally, the level of aftercare and ongoing monitoring required is often high, and the staff involved require regular training and support to ensure that a high-quality service is delivered.

The development of local institution-based protocols that harmonize with relevant national and international guidelines is strongly advised, as this provides a robust framework of standards and processes in which the service can operate.[2]

Patients should also be fully prepared for the block in the preoperative period (see Chapter 2) with a full explanation of the goals of such a treatment, other options and the warning signs of potential complications – paper-based or online resources are helpful and may help to improve the retention of information.[3]

Neuraxial blocks

Neuraxial blocks may be spinal, epidural or a combined spinal epidural (CSE). They provide high-quality analgesia in the perioperative period, but they require an advanced skillset for insertion and monitoring and can be associated with complications, though this is rare.[4]

A variety of devices and techniques have been developed to enable intraspinal drug delivery. They range from a single-shot injection through a specific needle to systems with external computer-controlled pumps that infuse drugs via a catheter, enabling longer-term management of pain. As with all interventional pain procedures, a comprehensive understanding of patient selection, the appropriate technical approaches and the equipment available, as well as the management of potential complications, is key.

Factors that may preclude a neuraxial technique include coagulopathy, infection (either bacteremia or at the site of insertion) and inability to tolerate hemodynamic change (sympathectomy may cause hypotension).

The degree of complexity and relative invasiveness of the technique adopted varies and the selection of the optimal approach is often influenced by multiple factors, some of which are outlined above.

In the perioperative period, most spinal blocks or epidurals are inserted before the surgical insult, using either an anatomic landmark technique or appropriate image guidance (such as ultrasound). The goal is to deliver the required drug into the desired space – this differs between techniques, with a spinal injection accessing the cerebrospinal fluid in the intrathecal space and an epidural-catheter technique involving infiltration through a catheter into the epidural space. It is important to appreciate the different anatomic sites used in the two approaches (Figure 6.1). A combined technique, CSE, may be used if both rapid onset of surgical anesthesia and prolonged analgesia are needed.

A detailed description of the differing methods and equipment used in inserting neuraxial blocks is beyond the remit of this text (see Further resources on page 59).

Peripheral nerve blocks

Peripheral nerve blocks may take the form of a single injection block, an indwelling catheter or an injection of a longer-acting local anesthetic formulation. The use of ultrasound guidance has revolutionized this technique. Combinations of blocks and systemic agents may facilitate true 'multimodal' analgesia.

Interest in the integration of local anesthetic blocks of peripheral nerves that innervate anatomic regions into the perioperative analgesic management plan has increased markedly. There are a number of reasons, including advances in ultrasound and block-needle technology, a desire to minimize (or even eliminate) the use of opioids in the perioperative period and continuing research into the relevant anatomy that facilitates the development of novel block approaches.

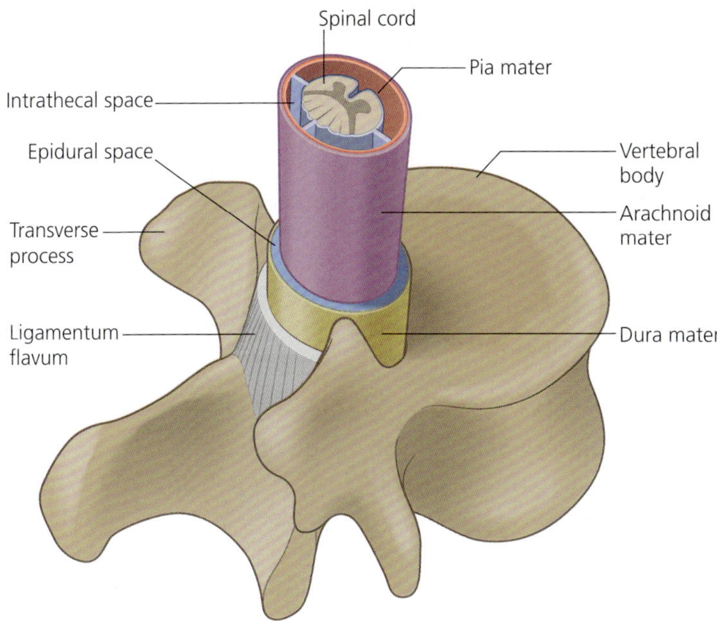

Figure 6.1 A lumbar vertebra showing the anatomy of the intrathecal and epidural spaces, which are relevant for spinal blocks and epidurals.

Single-shot blocks involve injecting local anesthetic in the perineural region, resulting in a time-limited reduction in sensation at the area innervated. Block duration can be extended by:

- increasing the dose of local anesthetic
- adding pharmacological adjuvants
- using novel products
- inserting indwelling catheters.

Dosing. There are ranges of local anesthetic concentrations and injectate volumes that can be utilized, and the concentration/volume selected will dictate the expected effect of a block. For example, a large volume of ropivacaine 0.5% used for an upper extremity nerve block would cause complete sensory and motor block appropriate for surgical anesthesia, whereas a smaller volume of ropivacaine 0.2% may produce incomplete numbness with motor sparing and would be more appropriate for postoperative pain.

Pharmacological adjuvants include the α-2 adrenoreceptor agonists clonidine and dexmedetomidine, the steroid dexamethasone and magnesium; the addition of these has been shown to increase the duration of analgesia by 2–8 hours.[5]

Novel products. Delivering bupivacaine in a liposomal preparation, where the active drug is encapsulated by lipid-based layers forming multiple honeycomb-like aqueous chambers, retards the delivery of the drug into the tissues, also prolonging its effect.[6] Infiltration with liposomal bupivacaine close to incisions has been demonstrated to reduce postoperative pain and the requirement for strong postoperative analgesia in a number of different surgical procedures, including abdominal and orthopedic procedures.[7,8]

Local anesthetic agents may also be combined with anti-inflammatory compounds to harness the complementary mechanisms of action of these drugs. One example is a preparation of bupivacaine and the NSAID meloxicam, which are combined in a polymer matrix that releases the drugs into the injection site over 72 hours. This dual-acting analgesic has been licensed for use in small to medium surgical wounds and represents an interesting addition to the postoperative analgesic armamentarium.

Local anesthetic infusion catheters have also been commonly adopted. Catheters may be inserted perioperatively in close proximity to the surgical wound (continuous wound infiltration), alongside relevant nerve plexi (perineural catheter analgesia) or within specific anatomic tissue planes.[9] The catheters used differ from those used for epidurals – they have microperforations along their length rather than fenestrations in their terminal portion. These microperforations allow local anesthetic to be infused for a greater distance, ensuring more extensive wound or nerve coverage. If combined with a portable pump, this technique can be used in ambulatory surgery.

Indwelling catheters represent a well-tolerated method of improving analgesia in the perioperative period. Theoretical complications include hematoma formation and local anesthetic toxicity. There is also the potential for wound infection, but this concern is not supported by clinical experience.[10,11]

The adoption of a new technique is influenced by the perceived benefit over existing approaches. When compared with epidural analgesia, preperitoneal catheters in abdominal surgery provide comparable analgesia, lower opioid consumption and hypotension and higher patient satisfaction.[12] This situation is mirrored in thoracotomy, where catheters placed in the paravertebral space provide comparable pain relief to traditional thoracic epidurals and may have a better side-effect profile.[13]

Topical agents

Local anesthetic may be applied topically, in the form of lidocaine gel or cream, ranging in strength from 1% to 4%, or in eutectic mixtures, such as lidocaine 2.5% and prilocaine 2.5%. Indications vary, as a topical agent can provide cutaneous analgesia prior to block placement in a sensitive patient (such as a child) or it can be applied several times a day in a thin layer in an attempt to provide ongoing analgesia for localized superficial pain.

Lidocaine 5% patches are most commonly used for pain associated with postherpetic neuralgia, but they can also be considered for use around surgical incisions or drains. Viscous lidocaine solutions can be useful in many instances of wound care. The solution should be applied 30 minutes before wound manipulation, to give adequate time for wound penetration.

Key points – non-systemic therapies

- The use of a local anesthetic block commonly forms an integral part of a multimodal approach to perioperative pain management.
- Neuraxial blocks are often viewed as the 'gold standard' for postoperative analgesia, but they may be associated with complications and require technical skills for their insertion and management.
- Advances in imaging techniques and equipment have recently made peripheral nerve or tissue plane blocks more popular.
- The duration of blocks may be prolonged by the addition of pharmacological adjuvants and the use of catheters and liposomal preparations of a local anesthetic drug.

References

1. Tucker GT. Pharmacokinetics of local anaesthetics. *Br J Anaesth* 1986;58:717–31.

2. Balasubramanian S, Baranowski AP, Barker C et al. *Core Standards for Pain Management Services in the UK*. Faculty of Pain Medicine of the Royal College of Anaesthetists, 2015.

3. Zarnegar R, Brown MRD, Henley M et al. Patient perceptions and recall of consent for regional anaesthesia compared with consent for surgery. *J R Soc Med* 2015;108: 451–6.

4. Cook TM, Counsell D, Wildsmith JAW. Major complications of central neuraxial block: report on the Third National Audit Project of the Royal College of Anaesthetists. *Br J Anaesth* 2009;102:179–90.

5. Desai N, Albrecht E, El-Boghdadly K. Perineural adjuncts for peripheral nerve block. *BJA Educ* 2019;19: 276–82.

6. Uskova A, O'Connor JE. Liposomal bupivacaine for regional anesthesia. *Curr Opin Anaesthesiol* 2015;28: 593–7.

7. Burnett A, Faley B, Nyirenda T, Bamboat ZM. Liposomal bupivacaine reduces narcotic use and time to flatus in a retrospective cohort of patients who underwent laparotomy. *Int J Surg* 2018;59:55–60.

8. Liu Y, Zeng JF, Zeng Y et al. Comprehensive comparison of liposomal bupivacaine with femoral nerve block for pain control following total knee arthroplasty: an updated systematic review and meta-analysis. *Orthop Surg* 2019; 11:943–53.

9. Scott NB. Wound infiltration for surgery. *Anaesthesia* 2010; 65(suppl 1):67–75.

10. Claroni C, Marcelli ME, Sofra MC et al. Preperitoneal continuous infusion of local anesthetics: what is the impact on surgical wound infections in humans? *Pain Med* 2016;17:582–9.

11. Zheng X, Feng X, Cai XJ. Effectiveness and safety of continuous wound infiltration for postoperative pain management after open gastrectomy. *World J Gastroenterol* 2016;22:1902–10.

12. Mungroop TH, Bond MJ, Lirk P et al. Preperitoneal or subcutaneous wound catheters as alternative for epidural analgesia in abdominal surgery: a systematic review and meta-analysis. *Ann Surg* 2019;269:252–60.

13. Ding X, Jin S, Niu X et al. A comparison of the analgesia efficacy and side effects of paravertebral compared with epidural blockade for thoracotomy: an updated meta-analysis. *PLoS One* 2014;9:e96233.

Further resources (neuraxial techniques)

Faculty of Pain Medicine of the Royal College of Anaesthetists. Clinical guidelines. www.fpm.ac.uk/standards-publications-workforce-guidelines-publications/clinical-guidelines, last accessed 5 August 2020.

Farag E, Mounir-Soliman L. *Brown's Atlas of Regional Anesthesia*, 5th edn. Elsevier, 2016.

New York School of Regional Anesthesia. Neuraxial techniques. www.nysora.com/techniques/neuraxial-and-perineuraxial-techniques, last accessed 5 August 2020.

7 Non-pharmacological management

Pain management in the perioperative period is important for a number of reasons. Poorly managed acute pain:

- is distressing for patients and their carers
- may contribute to increased length of stay
- increases the risk of postoperative morbidities, such as chest infections and deep vein thromboses.

Poorly managed acute pain may also increase the risk of the development of persistent postsurgical pain (see Chapter 9).

While pharmacological methods to control acute pain may be the first and most commonly considered approach, a range of non-pharmacological options are available. These may be considered both in isolation as well as integrated with more traditional methods. It is probably best to consider these from a biopsychosocial perspective, specifically the construct that pain (no matter its context) *impacts* and is *influenced by* the individual's biology, psychological wellbeing and social functioning. Hence, the benefit of addressing each facet of this model to achieve optimal pain control becomes clear. The major advantage of taking this approach is that pharmacological interventions can be avoided, or used at lower doses or for shorter duration, thereby reducing the risk of drug-associated harm.

Psychological interventions

Pain and psychological morbidity are inexorably interlinked – a patient with high levels of anxiety or pain-catastrophizing traits will commonly experience worse pain scores in the postoperative period than the norm. A patient experiencing severe, poorly controlled acute pain will understandably feel anxious – potentially establishing a negative spiral.

Although a number of approaches have been advocated, integrating psychological interventions into the perioperative pathway can prove challenging. The reasons include a lack of trained practitioners to deliver the care, financial costs and time pressures at the time of surgery (especially in oncology). Most interventions aim to normalize behavior; they include mindfulness, relaxation and breathing techniques and acceptance commitment therapy (ACT).[1] Many have been abridged in some way so that they can be delivered in a short timeframe. Despite the interest in these interventions, relatively limited evidence exists to support their use, though further work to better define their relevance is ongoing.[2]

An adjunct to psychological interventions is the concept of patient 'self-efficacy'.[3] The majority of patients want to recover from ill health rapidly, and better outcomes can be delivered by harnessing and supporting this desire. Examples of supporting self-efficacy include facilitating peer-to-peer support – for example, by organizing events where past patients can outline their experiences to current patients, answer any questions and provide reassurance, and running 'schools' attended by groups of patients before their surgery. At these events, the surgical journey can be explained in detail, misconceptions corrected and patients empowered to take ownership of some aspects of their care. These approaches form core components of the enhanced recovery after surgery (ERAS) approach and have become almost ubiquitous for some forms of surgery, such as arthroplasty.

Digital health solutions are also gaining traction in this field.

Acupuncture

Western medical acupuncture (WMA) involves placing fine acupuncture needles at various predetermined anatomic points for a period of time. It is distinct from traditional Chinese medicine acupuncture as it is considered to deliver its effects differently. WMA is known to have effects that are local (release of signaling molecules at the site of needling), segmental (alterations in the function of sensory nerves innervating the needled dermatome) and central (release of analgesic and anxiolytic signaling molecules within the central nervous system) (Figure 7.1).[4]

Acupuncture in the perioperative period is thought to provide analgesia, increase levels of energy and wellbeing and have anti-emetic effects.[5,6] The treatment modality is also popular among many patients, who view it as being 'natural' and complementary to their surgical treatment. Combining and integrating acupuncture with

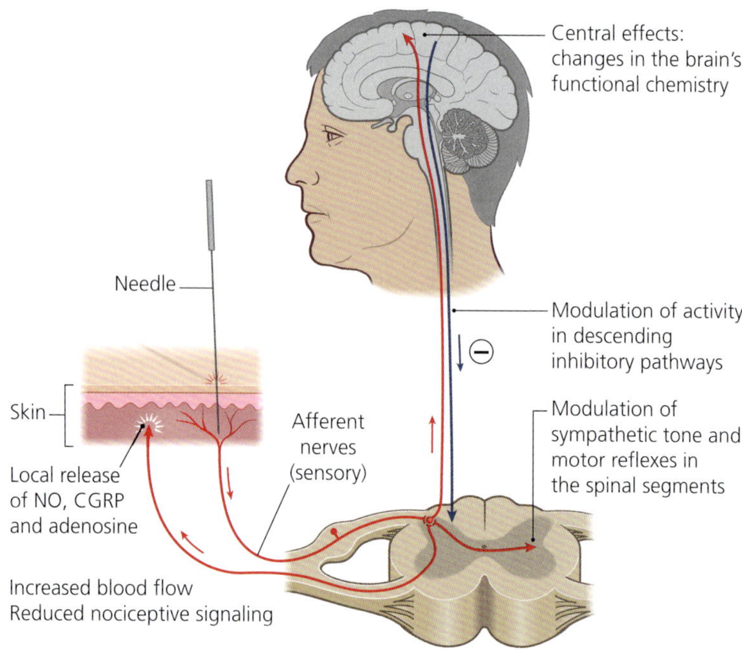

Figure 7.1 Western medical acupuncture appears to have local effects, segmental effects and central effects. CGRP, calcitonin gene-related peptide.

other approaches is likely to lead to the most benefit – this approach is taken in a number of centers across the globe.

Although the delivery of acupuncture to patients can potentially be resource intensive, the use of acupressure bands may provide a simple and cost-effective method to control postoperative nausea and vomiting.

Transcutaneous electrical nerve stimulation

TENS is a percutaneous non-interventional modality that uses the gate-control mechanism present in the spinal cord to modulate ascending pain signals. TENS equipment consists of an adhesive patch to apply to the skin and a small external generator box. Non-harmful electrical signals passing through the skin from the pad, via large diameter Aβ fibers, activate inhibitory interneurons within the dorsal horn of the spinal cord and enhance the descending inhibitory

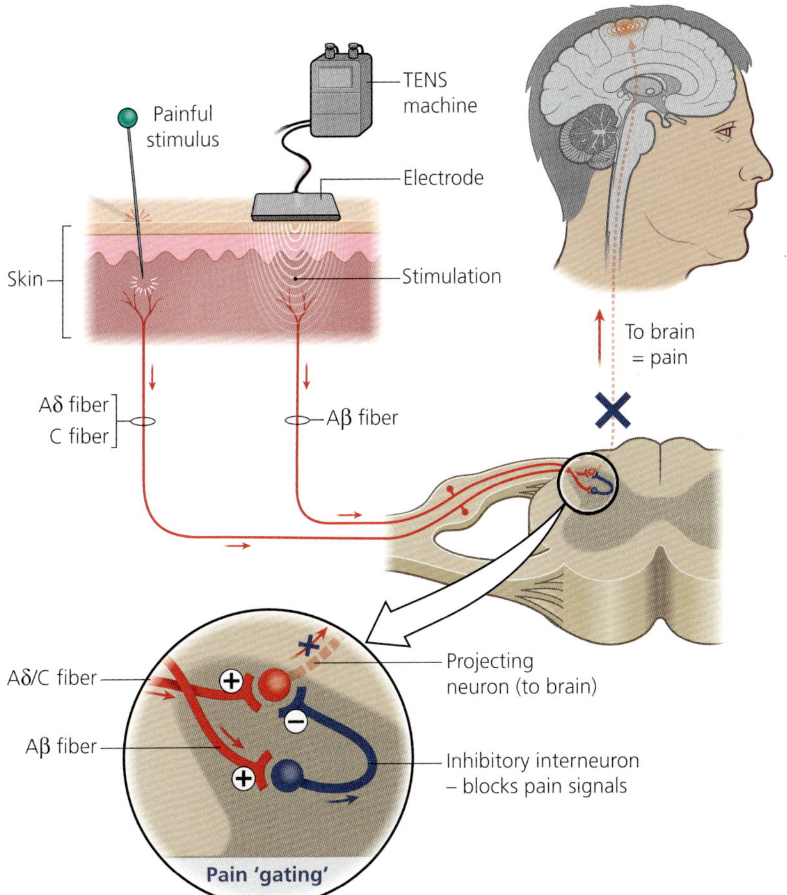

Figure 7.2 The proposed mechanism of action of TENS.

control pathways (Figure 7.2). These actions modulate pain signaling. In the periphery, TENS may alter the excitability of nociceptors, reducing afferent signals.[7]

Some evidence from systematic reviews exists to support the use of TENS in the perioperative period to help manage pain. TENS has been shown to be superior to placebo (no current) TENS for endpoints such as analgesic consumption and improvement in pain, pulmonary function and nausea and vomiting.[8] However, TENS would not be practicable for delirious patients or those with extensive wounds, such as those from burns.

Physical approaches

Encouraging early mobilization after surgery has multiple clearly defined benefits, including reduction in morbidity and shorter length of stay. Early (ideally, preoperative) engagement with physiotherapy permits a rehabilitative plan to be formulated in collaboration with the patient.[9] Regular review over the course of the admission enables changes in the rehabilitation plan to be made – this is a dynamic process, and alterations to the plan should not be viewed as failure. Alongside self-directed exercises, the use of thermal therapeutic interventions (hot and cold pads) can be beneficial – care should be taken when using these pads to avoid thermal injury.

Key points – non-pharmacological management

- A range of alternative non-pharmacological options are available for pain relief, which may be considered both in isolation and combined with analgesia.
- Interventions to address psychological issues are important – postoperative pain is commonly more severe in patients with anxiety or depression, and poorly controlled pain can be detrimental to a patient's psychological wellbeing.
- Physical interventions such as acupuncture, TENS and hot and cold pads can be useful adjuncts.
- Education and preparation of patients before their surgery may improve patient recovery times and reduce length of stay.

References

1. Azam MA, Weinrib AZ, Montbriand J et al. Acceptance and Commitment Therapy to manage pain and opioid use after major surgery: preliminary outcomes from the Toronto General Hospital Transitional Pain Service. *Can J Pain* 2017;1:37–49.

2. Nicholls JL, Azam MA, Burns LC et al. Psychological treatments for the management of postsurgical pain: a systematic review of randomized controlled trials. *Patient Relat Outcome Meas* 2018;9:49–64.

3. Nicholas MK. The pain self-efficacy questionnaire: taking pain into account. *Eur J Pain* 2007;11:153–63.

4. White A, Cummings M, Filshie J. *An Introduction to Western Medical Acupuncture*, 2nd edn. Elsevier, 2018.

5. Usichenko TI, Lehmann C, Ernst E. Auricular acupuncture for postoperative pain control: a systematic review of randomised clinical trials. *Anaesthesia* 2008; 63:1343–8.

6. Cheong KB, Zhang JP, Huang Y, Zhang ZJ. The effectiveness of acupuncture in prevention and treatment of postoperative nausea and vomiting – a systematic review and meta-analysis. *PLoS One* 2013;8:1–17.

7. Vance CGT, Dailey DL, Rakel BA, Sluka KA. Using TENS for pain control: the state of the evidence. *Pain Manag* 2014;4:197–209.

8. Johnson MI. Transcutaneous electrical nerve stimulation (TENS) as an adjunct for pain management in perioperative settings: a critical review. *Expert Rev Neurother* 2017; 17:1013–27.

9. Chou R, Gordon DB, de Leon-Casasola OA et al. Management of postoperative pain: a clinical practice guideline from the American Pain Society, the American Society of Regional Anesthesia and Pain Medicine, and the American Society of Anesthesiologists' Committee on Regional Anesthesia, Executive Committee, and Administrative Council. *J Pain* 2016;17:131–57.

8 Specific management strategies

When it comes to selecting a multimodal regimen (see Chapter 4), it is not a case of 'one size fits all'. Regimens should be thoughtfully tailored to an individual patient based on risk factors, patient preferences and the available evidence for specific procedure types. Involving the patient in formulating a perioperative pain management plan is widely accepted as beneficial.

Procedure-specific strategies

In 2016, guidelines on the management of postoperative pain were published on behalf of the American Pain Society, the American Society of Regional Anesthesia and Pain Medicine and the American Society of Anesthesiologists.[1] Table 8.1 summarizes reasonable options for some common procedures, drawn from these guidelines.

Looking at Table 8.1, all types of surgery have an identified role for opioids and routine use of NSAIDs and/or paracetamol for patients without a contraindication. NSAIDs are contraindicated in patients following coronary artery bypass grafting (CABG) surgery because of the increased risk of cardiovascular events. Some observation studies have revealed concerns regarding non-union following spinal fusion with high-dose NSAIDs and potential for anastomotic leakage after colorectal surgery. However, given the lack of high-quality evidence, it is reasonable to make decisions on a case-by-case basis, taking into account patient factors and surgical concerns.

Perioperative oral gabapentin/pregabalin and IV ketamine infusions are ubiquitously recommended as well, whereas agents like IV lidocaine have the best evidence for use following abdominal surgery.

Topical local anesthetics or the delivery of local anesthetic through regional or neuraxial techniques could be considered for all procedures as long as the agent can be appropriately targeted to the procedural site.

TABLE 8.1

Possible components of multimodal therapy for common types of surgery

Thoracotomy

Systemic

- Opioids*
- NSAIDs† ± paracetamol
- Gabapentin or pregabalin†
- Ketamine IV‡

Regional

- Paravertebral block

Neuraxial

- Epidural with LA (± opioid)
- Intrathecal opioid

Non-pharmacological

- Cognitive modalities
- TENS

Open laparotomy

Systemic

- Opioids*
- NSAIDs† ± paracetamol
- Gabapentin or pregabalin†
- Ketamine IV‡
- Lidocaine IV

Local/intra-articular/topical

- LA at incision
- Lidocaine, IV infusion

Regional

- Transversus abdominis plane block

Neuraxial

- Epidural with LA (± opioid)
- Intrathecal opioid

Non-pharmacological

- Cognitive modalities
- TENS

Total hip or knee replacement

Systemic

- Opioids*
- NSAIDs† ± paracetamol
- Gabapentin or pregabalin†
- Ketamine IV‡

Local/intra-articular/topical

- Intra-articular LA ± opioid

Regional

- Site-specific regional anesthetic technique with LA

Neuraxial

- Epidural with LA (± opioid)
- Intrathecal opioid

Non-pharmacological

- Cognitive modalities
- TENS

(CONTINUED)

TABLE 8.1 (CONTINUED)

Possible components of multimodal therapy for common types of surgery

Spinal fusion	
Systemic • Opioids* • Paracetamol§ • Gabapentin or pregabalin† • Ketamine IV‡ *Local/intra-articular/topical* • LA at incision	*Neuraxial* • Epidural with LA (± opioid) • Intrathecal opioid *Non-pharmacological* • Cognitive modalities • TENS
Cesarean section	
Systemic • Opioids* • NSAIDs† ± paracetamol *Local/intra-articular/topical* • LA at incision	*Regional* • Transversus abdominis plane block *Neuraxial* • Epidural with LA (± opioid) • Intrathecal opioid *Non-pharmacological* • Cognitive modalities • TENS
CABG	
Systemic • Opioids* • Paracetamol • Gabapentin or pregabalin† • Ketamine IV‡	*Non-pharmacological* • Cognitive modalities • TENS

Intra-articular, peripheral regional and neuraxial techniques are not typically used together.
*IV via PCA if parenteral route needed for more than a few hours and patient can understand the device and safety limitations.
†Can be given preoperatively.
‡Primarily consider for opioid-tolerant or otherwise complex patients.
§Adjunctive.
LA, local anesthetic.
From Chou et al. 2016.[1]

The inclusion of non-pharmacological strategies – cognitive modalities and TENS – should be expected as well. These generally present little to no patient risk.

Enhanced recovery after surgery

ERAS is an evidence-based multimodal and multidisciplinary approach to comprehensive perioperative care. Protocols include recommendations for pre-, intra- and postoperative care. They range from pre-admission nutritional support and smoking cessation to intraoperative fluid management and temperature control to multimodal opioid-sparing pain control facilitating earlier mobilization.[2,3] Overall goals include shortened hospital stays with reductions in complications and readmissions.[4]

Although the emphasis is not on pain control, published ERAS guidelines incorporate at least some recommendations on multimodal analgesia, opioids and regional/neuraxial approaches for specific procedures (see Useful resources, page 94).[5] All patients may be susceptible postoperatively to the sequelae of poorly controlled pain, which include delayed oral intake, delayed mobilization and prolonged hospitalization. These risks are in addition to the known adverse effects of opioid medications, which include nausea, ileus, respiratory depression and delirium.

Specific populations

Strategies for postoperative pain care should be adapted to individual groups, as well as to specific types of surgery.

Babies and children. The field of pediatric pain is considered its own specialty, but some general clinical considerations will be highlighted here.

Neonates and infants pose a particular challenge in terms of assessing pain.[6] Assessment tools include parameters such as behavior, crying, extremity tone, facial expression, vital signs, breathing pattern and consolability. This population also has special pharmacokinetic and pharmacodynamic considerations until 6–12 months of age.

Opioid medications should be dosed at 'one-quarter' to one-third of the recommended weight-based starting dose for children and titrated based on effect. Infants develop tolerance to opioids more quickly than older children, so dose adjustments may need to be made more often.[7]

Non-opioid medications may require longer or shorter dosing intervals, depending on metabolism.

Topical anesthetics such as lidocaine 2.5% and prilocaine 2.5% should be used when possible, keeping in mind that large or repeated doses are associated with methemoglobinemia, particularly in infants under 3 months of age.

Regional anesthetic techniques can be integral to postoperative pain management in infancy. A single-shot caudal epidural may suffice for analgesia for many outpatient procedures, such as hernia repair, or epidural catheters may be placed and tunneled for more intensive procedures, where a longer duration of action is likely to be needed. Conditions such as myelomeningocele may affect the ability to place a catheter.

Unlike in the adult population, placement of neuraxial and regional blocks is more commonly performed while infants and children are anesthetized, to improve cooperation with the procedure.

Patient-controlled anesthesia. As children age, they become better able to self-report pain. By 3–4 years of age, children can use pictorial representations to communicate pain intensity (see Chapter 3). By 6 years, many children can be taught to use a PCA device based on their interpretation of pain and understanding that they need to push the button before their pain becomes too severe. Screening and education should ensure that a parent does not push the PCA button on behalf of a sleeping child as this nullifies the inherent safety features of PCA.

Interestingly, younger children may not need as much opioid medication as older children, as pain seems to be more severe as patients age. For example, one study showed that children with a mean age of 5 years who received only ibuprofen after tonsillectomy reported less postoperative pain than children with a mean age of 8 years who received ibuprofen alone or ibuprofen with opioids.[8] Younger children also returned to their regular activity sooner.

As children reach adolescence, pain treatment regimens begin to mirror adult regimens. Unfortunately, this population is also at risk for ongoing opioid use as well as death from prescription-related overdose. Studies have shown persistent use of opioids in up to 4.8%

of opioid-naive patients aged 13–21 years prescribed opioids following surgery.[9] Risk factors include older age, female sex, previous substance use disorder, chronic pain, filling an opioid prescription preoperatively and long-term opioid use among family members.[10]

Older adults (65 years or older). Poorly controlled postoperative pain may contribute to adverse outcomes by contributing to cardiac ischemia by way of tachycardia and/or hypertension and delirium, particularly in patients with a significant level of frailty identified preoperatively.[11,12] However, pain is often undertreated in the elderly because of concerns that medication-related side effects will contribute to delirium, falls and confusion. The fact that the geriatric population is particularly susceptible to effects of polypharmacy complicates matters further. All these aspects can make it challenging to implement a multimodal regimen.

Systemic therapies. When initiating systemic therapies, knowledge of age-related physiological changes as well as pharmacokinetics and pharmacodynamics is important to make appropriate dose and timing adjustments for specific medications.[13] For example, given reduced renal clearance and glomerular filtration rate (GFR), NSAID doses should be reduced (7.5 mg ketorolac IV versus 15 mg in a younger adult, for example). Decreased hepatic function should prompt reduction of paracetamol dosing to a maximum of 3 g per 24 hours.

When prescribing medications that may affect sedation level or contribute to delirium, it is prudent to start one medication at a time to assess for effects. Low-potency opioids, such as oral tramadol or IV nalbuphine, should be considered in patients who do not seem to tolerate the effects of higher potency opioids.

Regional and neuraxial catheters that reduce the need for systemic therapies can be particularly helpful in the elderly. Epidural placement may be more challenging in patients with significant degenerative changes and sympathectomy may cause more pronounced hypotension than in a younger adult patient.

Individuals with underlying chronic pain. Treatment of acute pain that coexists with underlying chronic pain can be particularly challenging, especially in those with opioid tolerance. Some suggestions are given in Box 8.1.[1]

BOX 8.1

Managing procedural pain in the presence of chronic pain

- Thorough preoperative evaluation and counseling can help with expectation management
- It may be appropriate to delay an elective procedure if a patient has a pre-existing painful condition or mood disorder that is poorly controlled or untreated
- Emphasize that the goal of postoperative pain treatment is not to be 'pain free' but to reduce pain to a tolerable level to facilitate recovery (for example, participate in physical therapy, sleep adequately)
- Implement an appropriate multimodal pain regimen. Regional/ neuraxial approaches and IV ketamine may be particularly helpful in opioid-tolerant patients
- Standard doses of opioid medications should be tried before escalation; opioid-tolerant patients may require higher doses than a typical patient
- Long-acting opioids should be restarted at their usual doses as long as there are no concerns for sedation or respiratory depression. Short-acting opioids (oral or PCA) may be used in addition for the treatment of acute pain
- Make a specific plan for how the patient will taper medications back to their baseline dose and who will be responsible for prescribing medications. Treatment duration should not be longer for patients using long-term opioid therapy than for opioid-naive patients

Key points – specific management strategies

- Multimodal regimens should be tailored to an individual patient based on risk factors, patient preferences and the evidence available for specific procedure types.
- Many procedure-specific ERAS protocols have been published; these contain some guidance regarding multimodal analgesia and opioid-sparing techniques.
- Infants, young children and adolescents require different strategies for pain assessment, and there are specific pharmacological and treatment considerations for these groups.
- Dosing systemic therapies appropriately for the older adult requires knowledge of the physiological changes that occur with aging and the impact on pharmacokinetics and pharmacodynamics.
- Patients on chronic opioid therapy should have any long-acting medications restarted. They may require higher doses of opioids than typical patients, but they should not require longer durations.

References

1. Chou R, Gordon DB, de Leon-Casasola OA et al. Management of postoperative pain: a clinical practice guideline from the American Pain Society, the American Society of Regional Anesthesia and Pain Medicine, and the American Society of Anesthesiologists' Committee on Regional Anesthesia, Executive Committee, and Administrative Council. *J Pain* 2016;17:131–57.

2. Dietz N, Sharma M, Adams S et al. Enhanced Recovery After Surgery (ERAS) for spine surgery: a systematic review. *World Neurosurg* 2019;130: 415–26.

3. Lassen K, Soop M, Nygren J et al. Consensus review of optimal perioperative care in colorectal surgery: Enhanced Recovery After Surgery (ERAS) Group recommendations. *Arch Surg* 2009;144:961–9.

4. Ljungqvist O, Scott M, Fearon KC. Enhanced recovery after surgery: a review. *JAMA Surg* 2017;152:292–8.

5. Beverly A, Kaye AD, Ljungqvist O, Urman RD. Essential elements of multimodal analgesia in Enhanced Recovery After Surgery (ERAS) guidelines. *Anesthesiol Clin* 2017; 35:e115–43.

6. Ferland CE, Vega E, Ingelmo PM. Acute pain management in children: challenges and recent improvements. *Curr Opin Anaesthesiol* 2018;31: 327–32.

7. Friedrichsdorf SJ. Multimodal pediatric pain management (part 2). *Pain Manag* 2017;7:161–6.

8. Sowder JC, Gale CM, Henrichsen JL et al. Primary caregiver perception of pain control following pediatric adenotonsillectomy: a cross-sectional survey. *Otolaryngol Head Neck Surg* 2016;155:869–75.

9. Harbaugh CM, Lee JS, Hu HM et al. Persistent opioid use among pediatric patients after surgery. *Pediatrics* 2018; 141:e20172439.

10. Harbaugh CM, Lee JS, Chua KP et al. Association between long-term opioid use in family members and persistent opioid use after surgery among adolescents and young adults. *JAMA Surg* 2019;154:e185838.

11. Partridge JS, Harari D, Dhesi JK. Frailty in the older surgical patient: a review. *Age Ageing* 2012;41:142–7.

12. Chow WB, Rosenthal RA, Merkow RP et al. Optimal preoperative assessment of the geriatric surgical patient: a best practices guideline from the American College of Surgeons National Surgical Quality Improvement Program and the American Geriatrics Society. *J Am Coll Surg* 2012;215:453–66.

13. Setia S, Rooke AG. Perioperative care of elderly patients. In: Jackson MB, Mookherjee S, Hamlin NP, eds. *The Perioperative Medicine Consult Handbook*, 2nd edn. Springer, 2015:243–50.

9 Persistent postsurgical pain

The development of chronic pain after surgery – persistent postsurgical pain (PPSP) – is a relatively new concept. It is, however, an important condition and one that contributes significantly to the symptom burden of patients undergoing surgery. It can result in poor outcomes, negatively affecting a patient's quality of life and potentiating opioid misuse disorder.

PPSP remains poorly defined, but it is broadly recognized as being pain present (either continuously or arising de novo) for a minimum of 3 months after surgery.

To make the diagnosis, surgical and pre-existing causes of the pain should have been excluded.[1,2] The condition is common, with estimations of its prevalence ranging from 10% to 30% of all postsurgical patients.[3] Certain procedures are associated with a greater risk of developing PPSP – these include thoracotomy, cardiac surgery, breast surgery, limb amputation and hernia repair.[4] However, even relatively limited surgery, such as cutaneous melanoma removal, has been associated with the development of PPSP.[5]

Pathophysiology

The transition from acute pain to PPSP is complex and the mechanisms involved have not been fully delineated.[6] They do, however, reflect the complex and numerous processes triggered when injury to tissues occurs.

A huge number of neuron terminal fibers, cutaneous cells and immunocytes are present in the skin, and, following the noxious insult of surgery, these cells release myriad proinflammatory signaling molecules into both the local and locoregional environments.[7] In the periphery, these processes cause localized neuronal sensitization.[8] The resulting afferent barrage of nociceptive signaling leads to central sensitization, which manifests as enhanced nociceptive pathway neuronal functionality caused by increases in both membrane excitability and synaptic efficacy, as well as reduced inhibition.[9] This neuroplastic process depends on aberrant expression of ion channels on sensory neurons, resulting from alterations in gene expression,[10] and persistent neuroimmune interactions in the spinal cord and dorsal root ganglion (Figure 9.1).[11,12]

A prime example of PPSP is persistent pain following breast surgery, where a combination of neuropathic pain and sensory disturbance (commonly numbness in the distribution of the ipsilateral intercostobrachial nerve) results in hugely debilitating symptoms for those affected.

Risk factors

Despite PPSP undoubtedly being common, a proportion of patients undergo surgery without developing it, implying certain factors

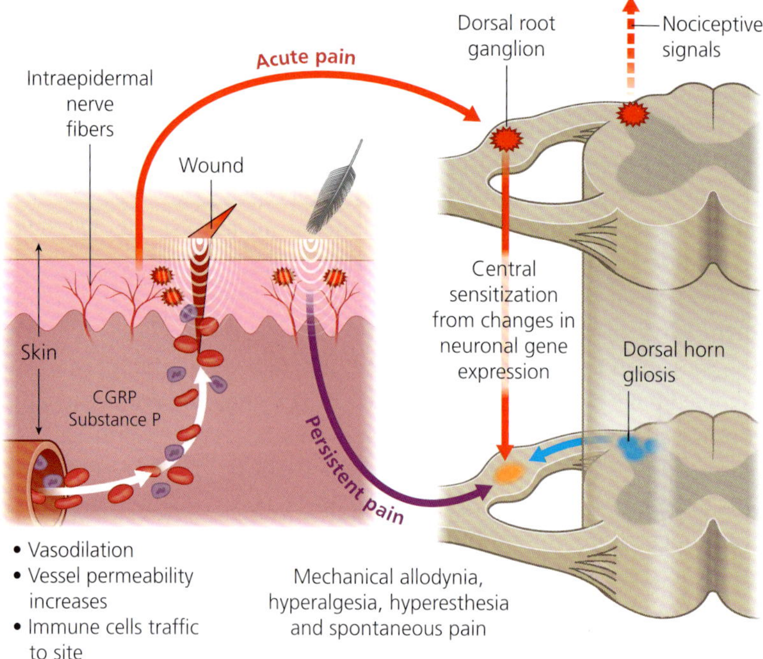

Figure 9.1 The proposed peripheral and central mechanisms that influence the transition from acute to persistent postsurgical pain. CGRP, calcitonin gene-related peptide.

predispose individuals to the condition. A number of important variables have been identified relating to both the patient and the surgery performed; these act as risk factors for the development of PPSP.

Surgery involving the division or prolonged retraction of nerves, such as thoracotomy or axillary clearance, is associated with higher rates of PPSP.[9] Extensive tissue disruption and damage, surgery duration of more than 3 hours,[13] and the use of surgical drains also appear to increase the risk of PPSP.[14]

Acute pain over the first 3–4 postoperative days increases the risk of transition to a persistent pain state,[15] and also predicts the development of PPSP.[14] This is likely related to increased peripheral and central neuronal sensitization.[16] Comparable neuroplastic influences may account for the fact that the presence and intensity of *preoperative* pain strongly predicts the occurrence of persistent pain after surgery.[17]

A variety of distinct patient factors have additionally been shown to contribute to an individual's risk profile for PPSP. Sex and age are important – with younger females at higher risk of pain chronicity[18] – as are genetic and epigenetic influences.[12] Psychological morbidity in the perioperative period is also important; anxiety, depression or the propensity to catastrophize renders patients at higher risk.[19]

Exposure to chemotherapy or radiotherapy around the time of surgery remains somewhat contentious as a risk factor – multiple studies have failed to demonstrate an association definitively.[20,21] However, certain chemotherapeutic agents are associated with an increased risk of peripheral neuropathy,[22] and work with laboratory models of PPSP shows a role for the transient receptor potential cation channel subfamily V member 1 (TRPV1) channel (the expression of which is increased in chemotherapy-induced peripheral neuropathy) in the potentiation of peripheral sensory nerve hypersensitivity following surgery.[23]

Predicting risk for developing PPSP is a relatively novel field, but it is attracting significant interest as the benefit of identifying modifiable factors in the perioperative period is clear. The majority of published research focuses on identifying those patients at high risk of developing severe acute postsurgical pain by either screening for known risk factors,[24] or using defined psychophysical tests, such as the patient's response to stereotyped painful stimuli in an experimental context.[25]

Work on predicting persistent pain following surgery has, in general, been surgery-type specific; for example, a tool has been produced that integrates patient and surgical factors during breast surgery, based on data from three distinct patient cohorts.[26]

Prevention and management

Because PPSP is relatively common, and because its development can be so detrimental to recovery, a number of preventive interventions have been investigated. These include so-called 'pre-emptive analgesia' – the administration of analgesic agents with the aim of pre-empting central sensitization, thereby reducing the risk of it occurring.

Several classes of drugs have been extensively investigated in the perioperative period, including the gabapentinoids pregabalin and gabapentin, and the NMDA receptor antagonist ketamine. However, the impact these agents have on the development of PPSP could be described at best as underwhelming, with limited conclusive data available to support their use.[27,28]

Further interest has focused on regional anesthetic techniques, including nerve blocks, neuraxial approaches such as spinal blocks and epidurals, and infiltration of the tissues with local anesthetics.[29] While for certain surgical approaches, thoracotomy for example, some evidence exists for benefit from specific procedures, such as an epidural, the findings of many of the studies are ambiguous and certainly not of an evidence level to support recommendations.

Added to the somewhat hazy evidence mix is the fact that the situation is dynamic with regard to regional anesthesia. The improved availability and quality of ultrasound machines means that the type and number of blocks that can be performed perioperatively is ever increasing and so the available options are expanding. One potential downside to this is that, because of the timing of PPSP (it occurs several months after surgery), there is little research conducted with new techniques to investigate the impact they have on the occurrence of PPSP.

When perioperative approaches to reduce PPSP risk are considered, the importance of routinely undertaking relatively simple measures is clear. These measures include:

- screening patients in the preoperative period for the presence of chronic pain or analgesic intake and for pre-existing psychological morbidity
- ensuring that patient expectations regarding perioperative pain are managed
- effectively controlling acute pain postoperatively.

Key points – persistent postsurgical pain

- PPSP is common, with prevalence estimates ranging from 10% to 30% of all postsurgical patients.
- PPSP results in poor surgical outcomes, negatively affecting patients' quality of life and potentiating opioid misuse disorder.
- PPSP is commonly associated with specific surgical procedures, such as breast surgery, thoracotomy, sternotomy and hernia repair.
- Some features of neuropathic pain occur with PPSP and the condition can prove challenging to treat.
- A number of risk factors for developing PPSP have been identified, including preoperative psychological morbidity and pain, surgical site, use of drains and severity of acute pain.

References

1. Levy N, Mills P, Rockett M. Post-surgical pain management: time for a paradigm shift. *Br J Anaesth* 2019;123:e182–6.

2. Werner MU, Kongsgaard UE. I. Defining persistent post-surgical pain: is an update required? *Br J Anaesth* 2014;113:1–4.

3. Bruce J, Quinlan J. Chronic post surgical pain. *Rev Pain* 2011;5:23–9.

4. Cregg R, Anwar S, Farquhar-Smith P. Persistent postsurgical pain. *Curr Opin Support Palliat Care* 2013;7:144–52.

5. Høimyr H, von Sperling ML, Rokkones KA et al. Persistent pain after surgery for cutaneous melanoma. *Clin J Pain* 2012;28:149–56.

6. Kalso E. IV. Persistent post-surgery pain: research agenda for mechanisms, prevention, and treatment. *Br J Anaesth* 2013;111:9–12.

7. Hou Q, Barr T, Gee L et al. Keratinocyte expression of calcitonin gene-related peptide β: implications for neuropathic and inflammatory pain mechanisms. *Pain* 2011;152: 2036–51.

8. Reichling DB, Green PG, Levine JD. The fundamental unit of pain is the cell. *Pain* 2013;154(suppl 1): 10.1016/j.pain.2013.05.037.

9. Kehlet H, Jensen TS, Woolf CJ. Persistent postsurgical pain: risk factors and prevention. *Lancet* 2006;367:1618–25.

10. Ji RR, Woolf CJ. Neuronal plasticity and signal transduction in nociceptive neurons: implications for the initiation and maintenance of pathological pain. *Neurobiol Dis* 2001;8:1–10.

11. Calvo M, Bennett DL. The mechanisms of microgliosis and pain following peripheral nerve injury. *Exp Neurol* 2012;234:271–82.

12. Richebé P, Capdevila X, Rivat C. Persistent postsurgical pain: pathophysiology and preventative pharmacologic considerations. *Anesthesiology* 2018;129:590–607.

13. Peters ML, Sommer M, de Rijke JM et al. Somatic and psychologic predictors of long-term unfavorable outcome after surgical intervention. *Ann Surg* 2007;245: 487–94.

14. Peng Z, Li H, Zhang C et al. A retrospective study of chronic post-surgical pain following thoracic surgery: prevalence, risk factors, incidence of neuropathic component, and impact on qualify of life. *PLoS One* 2014;9:e90014.

15. Perkins FM, Kehlet H. Chronic pain as an outcome of surgery. A review of predictive factors. *Anesthesiology* 2000;93:1123–33.

16. Katz J, Seltzer Z. Transition from acute to chronic postsurgical pain: risk factors and protective factors. *Expert Rev Neurother* 2009;9:723–44.

17. Tsirline VB, Colavita PD, Belyansky I et al. Preoperative pain is the strongest predictor of postoperative pain and diminished quality of life after ventral hernia repair. *Am Surg* 2013;79:829–36.

18. Liu SS, Buvanendran A, Rathmell JP et al. A cross-sectional survey on prevalence and risk factors for persistent postsurgical pain 1 year after total hip and knee replacement. *Reg Anesth Pain Med* 2012;37:415–22.

19. Belfer I, Schreiber KL, Shaffer JR et al. Persistent postmastectomy pain in breast cancer survivors: analysis of clinical, demographic, and psycho-social factors. *J Pain* 2013;14: 1185–95.

20. Andersen KG, Kehlet H. Persistent pain after breast cancer treatment: a critical review of risk factors and strategies for prevention. *J Pain* 2011;12:725–46.

21. Mejdahl MK, Andersen KG, Gärtner R et al. Persistent pain and sensory disturbances after treatment for breast cancer: six year nationwide follow-up study. *BMJ* 2013;346:f1865.

22. Brown M, Farquhar-Smith P. Pain in cancer survivors; filling in the gaps. *Br J Anaesth* 2017;119:723–36.

23. Barabas ME, Stucky CL. TRPV1, but not TRPA1, in primary sensory neurons contributes to cutaneous incision-mediated hypersensitivity. *Mol Pain* 2013;9:9.

24. Liu SS, Buvanendran A, Rathmell JP et al. Predictors for moderate to severe acute postoperative pain after total hip and knee replacement. *Int Orthop* 2012;36:2261–7.

25. Strulov L, Zimmer EZ, Granot M et al. Pain catastrophizing, response to experimental heat stimuli, and post-cesarean section pain. *J Pain* 2007;8:273–9.

26. Meretoja TJ, Andersen KG, Bruce J et al. Clinical prediction model and tool for assessing risk of persistent pain after breast cancer surgery. *J Clin Oncol* 2017;35:1660–7.

27. Chaparro LE, Smith SA, Moore RA et al. Pharmacotherapy for the prevention of chronic pain after surgery in adults. *Cochrane Database Syst Rev* 2013;2013:CD008307.

28. Martinez V, Pichard X, Fletcher D. Perioperative pregabalin administration does not prevent chronic postoperative pain: systematic review with a meta-analysis of randomized trials. *Pain* 2017;158:775–83.

29. Andreae MH, Andreae DA. Regional anaesthesia to prevent chronic pain after surgery: a Cochrane systematic review and meta-analysis. *Br J Anaesth* 2013;111:711–20.

10 Substance use disorder

By definition, substance use disorder (SUD) occurs when the use of one or more substances leads to clinically significant dysfunction, characterized by the compulsive use of substances, cravings, loss of control, and negative social consequences related to ongoing use. Substance use may lead to addiction, physical dependence or both.

There is still much to learn regarding the neurobiology of substance use, but there is well-supported evidence that disruption in the basal ganglia, extended amygdala and prefrontal cortex is key to the onset, development and maintenance of SUDs (Figure 10.1).[1] Each of these areas correlates to a different stage of the addiction cycle: binge/intoxication, withdrawal/negative affect and preoccupation/anticipation, respectively. A specific person may cycle through the stages over weeks to months, or even multiple times in a day, with each cycle resulting in continued changes in the brain through modulation of various neurotransmitters and neural circuits. The effects on the brain may persist even after substance use has stopped and it is unclear to what degree these changes can be reversed or how easily they can be reactivated.

Identification

It is essential to identify patients with SUD to safely provide perioperative pain care, given that both acute intoxication and/or withdrawal may complicate assessment. Perhaps more importantly, the specific type and severity of SUD will impact a patient's risk for overdose, misuse and diversion of opioids or other controlled substances on discharge from the hospital.

A thorough preoperative social history, including use of alcohol, tobacco and other drugs, should be obtained from all patients. Validated questionnaires such as the AUDIT-C (see www.mdcalc.com/audit-c-alcohol-use) may be used to screen for problematic alcohol use. For illicit substances, consider using a single-question screening tool such as, 'How many times in the past year have you used an illegal

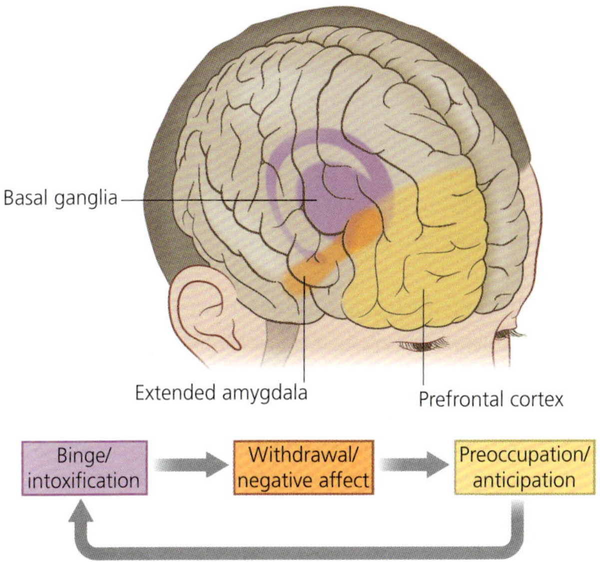

Figure 10.1 Brain regions associated with the three stages of addiction. The basal ganglia include the nucleus accumbens, which is involved in motivation and reward pathways, and the dorsal striatum, which is involved in habit forming. Addictive substances produce rewarding effects in the binge/intoxication stage of the cycle by activating the brain's dopamine and opioid signaling systems, while repeated activation contributes to habit forming. The extended amygdala is responsible for stress reactions, 'fight or flight' and negative emotions such as anxiety, irritability and depression. Activation of this area via neurotransmitters such as corticotropin-releasing factor and dynorphin, paired with reduced activity of the reward pathways in the basal ganglia are responsible for the negative feelings associated with withdrawal. Attempts to reduce these negative emotions contribute to compulsive substance use. The prefrontal cortex regulates executive function including organization of thoughts, decision making, time management, emotions and impulses. During the preoccupation/anticipation stage the prefrontal cortex is compromised as a person may become preoccupied with using a substance again after a period of abstinence ('craving'). Glutamate activity increases which, in turn, disrupts dopamine pathways. The end result is greater reactivity of habit-forming neural circuits with reduced inhibition of impulsive and compulsive substance seeking. Different substances affect each area of the brain in different ways depending on specific pharmacokinetics, but the general underlying principles are the same.

drug or a prescription medication for non-medical reasons?' and obtain additional history as appropriate.[2]

Referral to screening, brief intervention, and referral to treatment (SBIRT) services (USA) or the local drug and alcohol service (UK, via the general practitioner) should be recommended for any potential SUD, as well as referral to a methadone clinic or office-based addiction treatment (OBAT) program for patients with identified opioid use disorder (OUD).

The *Diagnostic and Statistical Manual of Mental Disorders* (fifth edition; DSM-5) criteria from the American Psychiatric Association can be useful for making an official diagnosis of SUD and/or OUD.[3] The criteria assess craving, tolerance and withdrawal, as well as the consequences of use. The level of SUD may be categorized as mild, moderate or severe depending on the number of criteria met. If an SUD is identified, the patient should be screened for relevant medical conditions, including hepatitis, cirrhosis, HIV, endocarditis, depression/anxiety and PTSD.[4]

Language

Regardless of who is obtaining patient history or making a diagnosis of SUD, non-judgmental and respectful language should be used with patients and other health professionals (Table 10.1). This encourages open and honest communication and reduces stigma regarding the diagnosis.[5]

Timing of surgery

For elective surgery, it is reasonable to postpone surgery for patients with newly identified uncontrolled SUD, given concerns for postoperative complications, including increased risk of infection, fall and overdose. This may not be possible for urgent or emergent cases, but hospitalization in general can serve as an opportunity to educate an individual on treatment options or even initiate treatment in medication-assisted therapy (MAT) for OUD.

Withdrawal syndromes

Understanding various withdrawal syndromes and their management is helpful when providing postoperative pain care (Table 10.2).[6]

TABLE 10.1

Preferred non-judgmental terminology

Preferred	Avoid
Substance use disorder	Substance abuse
Person/patient with SUD	Addict, drug user, IVDUer
Negative/positive urine drug test	Clean/dirty urine
In recovery/remission	Clean, sober
Treatment attempt	Treatment failure
Return to use	Relapse
Withdrawal	Dope sick, cold turkey

In the perioperative setting

In light of the ongoing opioid epidemic, medical providers are likely to come across patients with both treated and untreated OUD in the perioperative setting.[8,9] Methadone and buprenorphine–naloxone are two medications likely to be used in OUD.

Methadone is a µ-opioid receptor agonist and NMDA receptor antagonist. It has a variable and long elimination half-life of 24–48 hours, making it difficult to titrate rapidly. It is usually administered as a once-daily dose in solution form, with typical average doses of 80–100 mg. This contrasts with chronic pain dosing, which is in pill form, two to three times a day, with a usual total daily dose under 30 mg.

Buprenorphine–naloxone. Buprenorphine is a partial µ-opioid agonist. Naloxone is an opioid receptor antagonist. The combination is prescribed as a sublingual tab or film given either daily or divided into two to four doses per day. Buprenorphine is the primary active medication, as naloxone is poorly absorbed sublingually and is intended as a deterrent for misuse by IV injection. Like methadone, buprenorphine has a variable and long elimination half-life, usually 24–42 hours.

TABLE 10.2

Withdrawal syndromes, management and effect on postoperative care

Withdrawal syndrome	Management	Special considerations in postoperative care
Tobacco		
• Irritability, restlessness, nausea, sweating • Peaks within 3 days of last use	• Nicotine replacement (patch, gum/lozenge) • Varenicline • Bupropion	• Nicotine, regardless of form, may impact wound and bone healing • Consultation with surgeon advised
Alcohol		
• Restlessness, agitation, nausea, increased blood pressure, tremor, delirium, seizures • Begins 6–24 hours after last use	• Monitoring • Symptom-triggered treatment with benzodiazepines or phenobarbital, based on Clinical Institute Withdrawal Assessment for Alcohol (CIWA)	• Delirium related to withdrawal may be difficult to discern from other causes • Gabapentin may be useful for pain and withdrawal • Adjust doses of medications such as paracetamol as risk of underlying liver dysfunction • Assess for risk of gastrointestinal bleed prior to initiating NSAIDs

Opioids		
• Tachycardia, hypertension, enlarged pupils, diaphoresis, abdominal cramping, nausea, diarrhea, muscle pain • Presentation and duration depends on opioid used	• Consider initiating methadone (20–40 mg/24 hours) or buprenorphine–naloxone • Manage symptoms with, for example, clonidine, loperamide, ondansetron	• Opioid tolerance emphasizes the importance of a multimodal approach to pain • Adjust doses of medications such as paracetamol if concern for hepatitis C • Manage discharge sensitively to engage patients in MAT and minimize opioid prescriptions if there is concern for misuse or diversion • Discharge with naloxone
Benzodiazepines		
• Irritability, sleep disturbance, anxiety, tremors, delirium, seizures • Presentation depends on duration of action and chronicity of benzodiazepine used (hours to weeks)	• Treat with slow taper of benzodiazepines based on patient's history	• Concomitant use of benzodiazepines and opioids increases risk of respiratory depression

(CONTINUED)

TABLE 10.2 (CONTINUED)

Withdrawal syndromes, management and effect on postoperative care

Withdrawal syndrome	Management	Special considerations in postoperative care
Stimulants (methamphetamine, cocaine)		
• Fatigue, sleepiness, anxiety, depression, increased appetite • Typically presents several hours after last use	• Withdrawal not typically medically complex or life-threatening	• Catecholamine depletion may affect anesthetic management • Sedation may limit ability to use opioids, gabapentinoids or other medications with side effect of sedation • With IV use, patients may be at risk for hepatitis C • Patients may be at risk for misuse or diversion of opioids on discharge
Marijuana		
• Irritability, restlessness, sweating • Onset within hours of last use	• Withdrawal not typically medically complex • Treat symptoms as needed • Limited and inconsistent evidence to support pharmacological replacement with medications such as dronabinol	• Pharmacological interactions are poorly understood, though significant chronic use seems to increase the need for fentanyl, midazolam and propofol; opioid tolerance may be increased[7] • It is unclear whether cannabis products have a future role as an adjunct in pain management

Buprenorphine products without the naloxone component exist and are primarily used in pregnancy because the effects of naloxone on the fetus and in pain are unknown. Doses of buprenorphine in OUD vary widely, often ranging from 8 mg to 24 mg. In chronic pain, doses are typically lower: 0.5 mg three times a day, for example.

MAT with methadone and buprenorphine–naloxone can be very effective in treating OUD, particularly in combination with counseling and behavioral therapy. MAT helps normalize brain chemistry and relieve physiological cravings, while also blocking the reward effects of opioid use on the brain.

Patients receiving OUD treatment.

With methadone. The methadone dose should be confirmed with the patient's methadone clinic and the dose should be continued. Postsurgical acute pain may then be treated with additional short-acting opioids.

With buprenorphine–naloxone. The dose should be verified through a prescription-monitoring program and/or the patient's pharmacy/prescriber. Strong consideration should be given to continuing buprenorphine–naloxone throughout the entire perioperative period.[10]

Buprenorphine is known to have a very high affinity for opioid receptors. As a consequence, patients receiving buprenorphine have a reputation for resistance to pain management with traditional full opioid agonists. Because of this, some providers advocate stopping buprenorphine products 24–72 hours preoperatively and bridging with short-acting opioids. However, this practice can destabilize a patient with OUD and prompt them to return to use. By using a multimodal pain plan and other high-affinity opioids, such as hydromorphone and fentanyl, acute pain can be successfully treated in patients using buprenorphine–naloxone, even after major surgery, making continuation reasonable.

For patients at very high risk, a temporarily increased dose of buprenorphine–naloxone can be used for acute pain treatment. Otherwise, short-acting opioids such as hydromorphone and oxycodone can be given on an as-needed basis in addition to regular doses of buprenorphine–naloxone.

With extended-release naltrexone. For these patients, it is preferable to delay elective surgeries for 30 days after the last administered dose.

Patients not receiving OUD treatment. Postsurgical inpatients with identified OUD who are not engaged in treatment should be encouraged to consider methadone or buprenorphine–naloxone, as it is very challenging to treat acute pain if underlying opioid needs are not being met. Treatment options should be based on patient preference as well as access to care, as attending a methadone clinic for daily dosing may not be feasible for all patients.

Methadone may be started at a once-daily oral dose of 20–40 mg if withdrawal symptoms are present. If there is concern for sedation or other side effects in a medically complex patient, methadone may be started in divided doses, such as 10 mg orally every 8 hours. Divided doses may also take advantage of the typical 6–8-hour analgesic window associated with methadone, even if pain relief is not its primary purpose. Acutely, these low doses of methadone should mitigate the majority of withdrawal symptoms, but over time the dose may need to be increased to address cravings.[11]

Buprenorphine–naloxone can be more challenging to start in the perioperative setting. If a patient is able to tolerate a period of 8–12 hours without any opioid medication for their acute pain, they may be able to proceed with a traditional buprenorphine–naloxone induction. If buprenorphine–naloxone is initiated too soon after receiving other full opioid agonists, withdrawal can be precipitated, as the buprenorphine displaces other opioids from receptors.

Another method of initiating buprenorphine is through 'micro-induction': small amounts of buprenorphine are introduced (starting with 0.5 mg buprenorphine daily) and gradually increased in frequency and dose, typically over 5 days.[12] As buprenorphine reaches a steady state and other short-acting opioids continue to be tapered, doses of buprenorphine can be more liberally increased without concern for precipitating withdrawal.

Before initiating therapy with methadone or buprenorphine–naloxone, an electrocardiogram (ECG) should be obtained, because of the risk of QT prolongation. Healthcare providers should facilitate outpatient follow-up at a methadone clinic for an intake appointment (in the USA, by law, methadone can be dispensed only through an opioid treatment program certified by the Substance Abuse and Mental Health Services Administration [SAMHSA]) or OBAT clinic for continued prescribing of buprenorphine–naloxone (prescribers must have specific training to prescribe for addiction). Even if a patient chooses not to engage in long-term treatment for OUD, initiating treatment in the hospital has been shown to reduce the risk of opioid overdose on discharge.

Discharge planning

Whether a patient has a diagnosed SUD/OUD or is opioid naive, care should be taken to develop a discharge plan that encourages patients to discontinue opioid medication for acute pain within an appropriate period of time based on the type of surgery. Further, patients should not be provided with more medication than necessary.[13] Patients undergoing minor procedures may require minimal to no opioid medications, whereas patients undergoing major spine surgery may require 3–6 weeks of opioid management.[14]

Research indicates that doses of opioid medications provided postoperatively are less predictive of persistent opioid use after surgery than duration of initial therapy.[15] Use of tamper-resistant formulations of opioid medications, such as those that form viscous substances or gel matrices when manipulated, should be considered as a deterrent for misuse or diversion. All patients should be given information on tapering of opioid medications, risks of opioid therapy and safe disposal of excess medication.

Key points – substance use disorder

- SUD refers to the use of one or more substances that leads to clinically significant dysfunction, characterized by compulsive use of substances, cravings, loss of control and negative social consequences related to ongoing use.
- There is a strong neurobiological basis for SUD involving regulation by the basal ganglia, extended amygdala and prefrontal cortex, which correlate with three stages of addiction (binge/intoxication, withdrawal/negative affect and preoccupation/anticipation).
- Health professionals should obtain a thorough and accurate social history in a non-judgmental way to identify potential SUDs and refer for appropriate treatment.
- Treatment of OUD with methadone or buprenorphine–naloxone can be important in reducing perioperative risks, such as infection or overdose, and improving acute pain control. Pain is challenging to treat if a patient's underlying opioid needs are not being met.

References

1. Substance Abuse and Mental Health Services Administration (US), and Office of the Surgeon General (US). The neurobiology of substance use, misuse, and addiction. In: *Facing Addiction in America: The Surgeon General's Report on Alcohol, Drugs, and Health*. Reports of the Surgeon General. US Department of Health and Human Services, 2016. www.ncbi.nlm.nih.gov/books/NBK42485, last accessed 20 July 2020.

2. Smith PC, Schmidt SM, Allensworth-Davies D, Saitz R. A single-question screening test for drug use in primary care. *Arch Intern Med* 2010;170:1155–60.

3. American Psychiatric Association. Substance-related and addictive disorders. In: *Diagnostic and Statistical Manual of Mental Disorders*, 5th edn. APA, 2013. doi.org/10.1176/appi.books.9780890425596.dsm05.

4. Marschall KE, Hines RL. Psychiatric disease, substance abuse, and drug overdose. In: *Stoelting's Anesthesia and Co-Existing Disease*, 7th edn. Elsevier, 2017.

5. van Boekel LC, Brouwers EP, van Weeghel J, Garretsen HF. Stigma among health professionals towards patients with substance use disorders and its consequences for healthcare delivery: systematic review. *Drug Alcohol Depend* 2013;131:23–35.

6. Levitt DS, Klein JW. Substance use disorders. In: Jackson MB, Huang R, Kaplan E, Mookherjee S, eds. *The Perioperative Medicine Consult Handbook*, 3rd edn. Springer, 2020:371–80.

7. Twardowski MA, Link MM, Twardowski NM. Effects of cannabis use on sedation requirements for endoscopic procedures. *J Am Osteopath Assoc* 2019;10.7556/jaoa.2019.052.

8. Ward EN, Quaye AN, Wilens TE. Opioid use disorders: perioperative management of a special population. *Anesth Analg* 2018;127:539–47.

9. Quinlan J, Cox F. Acute pain management in patients with drug dependence syndrome. *Pain Rep* 2017;2:e611.

10. Acampora GA, Nisavic M, Zhang Y. Perioperative buprenorphine continuous maintenance and administration simultaneous with full opioid agonist: patient priority at the interface between medical disciplines. *J Clin Psychiatry* 2020;81:19com12810.

11. Dale RC, Metcalf CL, Langford DJ et al. An Acute Pain Service experience initiating methadone for opioid use disorder in hospitalized patients with acute pain. *J Opioid Manag* 2019;15:275–83.

12. Klaire S, Zivanovic R, Barbic SP et al. Rapid micro-induction of buprenorphine/naloxone for opioid use disorder in an inpatient setting: a case series. *Am J Addict* 2019; 28:262–5.

13. Hill MV, McMahon ML, Stucke RS, Barth RJ Jr. Wide variation and excessive dosage of opioid prescriptions for common general surgical procedures. *Ann Surg* 2017;265:709–14.

14. Bree R. Supplemental guidance on prescribing opioids for postoperative pain. www.breecollaborative.org/wp-content/uploads/Supplemental-Bree-AMDG-Postop-pain-18–0718.pdf, last accessed 25 June 2020.

15. Brummett CM, Waljee JF, Goesling J et al. New persistent opioid use after minor and major surgical procedures in US adults. *JAMA Surg* 2017;152:e170504.

Useful resources

Organizations

American Academy of Pain Medicine
painmed.org

American Society of Regional Anesthesia and Pain Medicine
www.asra.com

Australian Pain Society
www.apsoc.org.au

Australian and New Zealand College of Anaesthetists & Faculty of Pain Medicine
fpm.anzca.edu.au

British Pain Society
www.britishpainsociety.org

Centers for Disease Control and Prevention
www.cdc.gov/acute-pain/postsurgical-pain/index.html

European Society of Regional Anaesthesia and Pain Therapy (ESRA)
esraeurope.org

ERAS Society
erassociety.org

Faculty of Pain Medicine of the Royal College of Anaesthetists
fpm.ac.uk

International Association for the Study of Pain (IASP)
www.iasp-pain.org

New York School of Regional Anesthesia (NYSORA)
www.nysora.com

Guidelines

Chou R, Gordon DB, de Leon-Casasola OA et al. Management of postoperative pain: a clinical practice guideline from the American Pain Society, the American Society of Regional Anesthesia and Pain Medicine, and the American Society of Anesthesiologists' Committee on Regional Anesthesia, Executive Committee, and Administrative Council. *J Pain* 2016;17:131–57.

ERAS Society guidelines

Each institution or surgical center may choose to implement all or part of the guidelines as part of their local perioperative treatment. Additionally, some institutions have created pathways for other procedures such as major spine surgery or extremity amputations, which also reflect the available evidence in pain treatment.

Guidelines are available from erassociety.org/guidelines/list-of-guidelines, and include:

- Colonic resection 2012
- Rectal/pelvic resection 2012
- Cystectomy 2013
- Gastric resection 2014
- Bariatric surgery 2016
- Liver surgery 2016
- Head and neck cancer surgery 2016
- Breast reconstruction 2017
- Thoracic noncardiac surgery 2018
- Esophageal resection 2018
- Cesarean delivery (parts 1–3) 2018
- Colorectal surgery 2018
- Hip and knee replacement 2019
- Cardiac surgery 2019
- Major gynecologic/oncological surgery 2019
- Pancreaticoduodenectomy 2020

Prospect guidelines

Prospect (**pro**cedure **spec**ific postoperative pain managemen**t**), a group of surgeons and anesthesiologists, provides a clinical-decision-support service to improve the management of postoperative pain on a procedure-specific basis. Guidelines are available at esraeurope.org/prospect

Faculty of Pain Medicine Core Standards for Pain Management Services (CSPMS)

The CSPMS is a collaborative multidisciplinary publication providing a robust reference source for the planning and delivery of pain management services in the UK. Core standards are available at fpm.ac.uk/standards-publications-workforce/core-standards

Index